DEPRESSION TO HAPPINESS II

101 Nutrition and Lifestyle Secrets For Health and Happiness

By Timothy Baumann, CHC

Published by Wellness For Life Network, LLC
Ogden, Utah 84403

Visit our website at www.depressiontohappiness.com

10 9 8 7 6 5 4 3 2 1

Cover design by Timothy Baumann

ISBN: 978-0-9976187-1-6

Dedication

This book is dedicated to you, my wonderful and beautiful wife.

You are my motivation behind all I do.

Thank you for supporting me, once again, in another of my wild ideas.

You struggle with many health issues and have done so for most of your life. Together we have faced many trials and obstacles.

I strive to bring all the peace and comfort I can into your life.

May you find peace and happiness as we continue to travel through this life and the eternities – together.

DISCLAIMER

None of the information contained within this book has been approved by the Food and Drug Administration. Also consult with your health professional before you change your eating habits or embark on a new exercise routine. This book makes no claims to diagnose or cure any mental or physical maladies. We make no claims to any outcomes nor guarantee specific results.

Published by Wellness For Life Network, LLC
Ogden, Utah 84403

ACKNOWLEDGEMENTS

I need to acknowledge my parents, Edward and Sandra Baumann, who did a great job in raising me, their oldest child. I kindly joke that since I was the oldest of 5 children; I was the 'experiment' and that I along with my next two younger brothers, help "wear down my parents" because the youngest brother and sister sure were spoiled. Thanks again mom and dad for your support. Thank you mom for proof reading this book and correcting all my errors.

My nutrition and health coaching education came from the Institute of Integrated Nutrition (IIN) and Joshua Rosenthal. It was there that I first learned about biodiversity and that 'one man's food is another man's poison'. It was there that I also learned about Primary Foods and Secondary Foods. Primary Foods are foods that you do not eat but are essential for good health and Secondary Foods are the foods that you do eat. Both Foods have to be in balance for great health.

Lastly I need to acknowledge all the other health coaches, fellow IIN students and other alternative health practitioners who do a wonderful job in helping others regain and maintain their health using nutrition and alternative methods. I have learned so much from all of you. You give me courage to press on and follow in your footsteps of helping others.

TABLE OF CONTENTS

Maybe

PREFACE

Depression To Happiness II is a very condensed version of a complete holistic program that I put together to help individuals who suffer from symptom of depression and anxiety. It is called *Depression To Happiness – The 100 Day Challenge*. (More information can be found at www.depressiontohappiness.com/the100daychallenge)

I was motivated to write this book and The 100 Day Challenge because of my wife and some of her family members. A number of years ago my mother-in-law committed suicide and a few years later my brother-in-law committed suicide. Well luck would have it, my wife became depressed. I knew I had to do something or she might be the next one in her family to commit suicide.

I went to nutrition school for a year and then spent two years researching for natural, holistic ways to dealing with depression symptoms. She tried an anti-depressant and did not like the side effects or how they made her feel. So she went off the medication. In my research I found a supplement that has a 20 year track record of helping with depression and anxiety symptoms. She tried it and it really seemed to help her. Next was the lifestyle changes and healthy eating.

Depression To Happiness II – 101 Nutrition and Lifestyle Secrets For Health and Happiness is a collection of all the different tips, secrets and action items that can and will help diminish or eliminate depression and anxiety symptoms. You get just a little information on each secret and an action item.

The secret to success is in the action items. The idea is to read the book all the way through. Then each week work on implementing each action item and making that tip part of your daily life. Each action item is simple and easy to implement. Please don't knock any of the tips. They work and I challenge you to try each one. The proof is in the pudding.

The sole purpose of this book is to give you some ideas and simple action steps to improve your overall health. When your body is given the right nutrition, your body and brain will be healthy and will function properly. When it comes down to it, most all diseases and mood disorders can be improved or eliminated with proper nutrition and lifestyle changes. Try these 101 secrets and you will find the journey to peace and happiness quite enjoyable.

Happiness is all about the journey, not the destination.

INTRODUCTION

THE HAPPINESS JOURNEY

"For a long time it seemed to me that life was about to begin - real life. But there was always some obstacle in the way, something to be gotten through first, some unfinished business, time to still be served, a debt to be paid.

"Then life would begin. At last it dawned on me that these obstacles were my life.

"This perspective has helped me to see that there is <u>no way TO</u> happiness. Happiness <u>IS the way</u>.

So, treasure every moment that you have. And treasure it more because you shared it with someone special, special enough to spend your time and remember that time waits for no one.

So stop waiting
until you finish school,
until you go back to school,
until you lose ten pounds,
until you gain ten pounds,
until you have kids,
until your kids leave the house,
until you start work,

until you retire,
until you get married,
until you get divorced,
until Friday night,
until Sunday morning,
until you get a new car or home,
until your car or home is paid off,
until spring,
until summer,
until fall,
until winter,
until you are off welfare,
until the first or fifteenth,
until your song comes on,
until you've had a drink,
until you've sobered up,
until you die,
until you are born again
to decide that there is no better time than right now to
be happy.

Happiness is a journey, not a destination.
--Alfred D. Souza

Health and Happiness is the pursuit of most people in the world today. Unfortunately many people cannot find this allusive feeling. Why can't many people find real health and happiness? Here is something to think about —

INSANITY: Doing the same thing over and over and expecting a different result.

SADNESS: Staying on the same lifestyle path and expecting happiness.

HAPPINESS: The Happiness Journey requires you to change the path you are on by making lifestyle changes.

So if you want to enjoy the fruits of the journey to happiness you must make some changes. These changes do not have to be giant steps. Just the opposite is true. You only need to make consistent, small, and daily changes. If you do, one day you will find that you are on a different path, one that will lead you on the happiness journey.

The body, mind and soul must have all the proper nutrients to obtain and maintain good health in order to be happy. These nutrients are found in two main food groups – **Primary Foods** and **Secondary Foods**.

- _PRIMARY FOODS_: Keep in mind that not all nutrients come from the food we eat. These are foods that we do not eat. These are also considered Lifestyle Choices. The following fall into this category – **Exercise, Relationships, Careers and Spirituality**. If these areas in your life are missing or they are weak, you are not going to be getting the nutrition you need AND these 4 areas are causing you stress instead of strength.

- <u>SECONDARY FOODS:</u> These are the foods you do eat and drink. These are foods that provide most of the different nutrients that your body needs to grow and maintain good health. They provide nutrients such as Vitamins, Minerals, Micro and Macro Nutrients, Proteins, Carbohydrates, etc. Without adequate levels of all these different nutrients your body and mind will suffer.

This book is a list of 101 secret tips to incorporate into your daily life to help improve your physical health, your mental health and your spiritual or soul's health.

This book is **NOT** an exhaustive study of each tip. They are just that, tips to plant healthy seeds in your mind. It is up to you to fully research each tip and see if it applies to you and how you can fit it into your life.

I cannot guarantee results. But I can tell you that those who put forth the effort to apply as many of these tips into their lives as possible, have seen great results. I am not diagnosing nor giving medical advice, nor do I promote these tips as a cure for any mental or physical disease. But I will make a note that these tips have helped many people with mood disorders such as depression and anxiety. They have helped people with physical and spiritual disorders. I also want you to know that there have been studies done on most all of these tips so there is sound scientific backing for these tips. You will find that this is true, if you will do a little research.

Again, this is not an in-depth study on each tip, but you are given enough information to develop an understanding of the importance of the tip in your diet and your lifestyle.

Part of each tip is an action item. The real secret is in doing the action items. The evidence is in the results of doing the action items. In other words, do the action items and you will see the results.

Baseline Evaluation

Before you get started you need to first set a baseline for each of the major areas in your life. You need to really know where you need to focus most of your time and energy. So to do this you will need to go to the resource section at the end of the book and copy the "Bicycle Of Life" or the "Wheels of Life" as seen below.

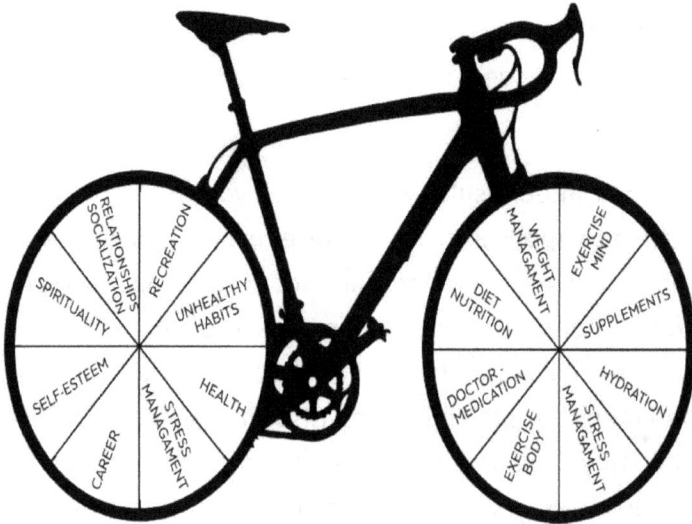

LIFE: PRIMARY WHEEL   **HEALTH: SECONDARY WHEEL**

Instructions:

For each section on each wheel, you need to ask yourself, **'How satisfied am I with how things are going with section _____ in my life?'** The outer rim of the tire is a 10 and the hub (center) of the wheel is a 0.

Place a dot along the line (spoke) where you are in each category. When it comes to the Stress Management there are two sections, one on each wheel. I want you to think about stress as it relates to the other areas of that particular wheel, not as a whole. So in the Primary Wheel think about stress as it relates to your relationships, career, your spirituality or the other sections of that wheel.

With the Secondary Wheel, evaluate your stress when it comes to your health, weight, mind and body, etc. Now take a look at your stress ratings for each wheel. You may find that most of your stress is related to your primary foods or your health. You may also find that whichever wheel has the lowest satisfaction rating for stress will also have some of the lowest ratings in some of the other sections. This may indicate which areas are causing you the most stress and therefore needs the most work. Now connect all the dots.

How round are your wheels? How smooth is your ride in life?

Keep one thing in mind. We are looking for smooth wheels NOT perfect 10's in each area.

This will now be your baseline. At the end of the 101 steps you will repeat the process to see just how far you have traveled on your Happiness Journey.

One last thing – before changing your diet or including exercise, please consult with a medical professional.

Enjoy the tips and enjoy the journey to better health and happiness!

PART 1 - PRIMARY FOODS

"Food is more than what you find on your plate. Healthy relationships, regular physical activity, a fulfilling career and a spiritual practice can fill your soul and satisfy your hunger for life. When primary food is balanced and satiated, your life feeds you, making what you eat secondary".

The Founder of Institute of Integrative Nutrition, Joshua Rosenthal

Joshua Rosenthal also said, *"We hunger for play, touch, romance, intimacy, love, achievement, success, art, music, self-expression, leadership, excitement, adventure and spirituality. All of these elements are essential forms of nourishment. The extent to which we are able to incorporate them determines how enjoyable and worthwhile our lives feel."*

1. SELF TALK

Self-talk is that conversation that goes on within your inner self. It is that inner voice in your mind that says stuff that you don't necessarily say out loud. Much of the time this self-talk happens and you don't even realize it going on. It can be a quiet discussion going on in the background of your mind. Just know that what you say in your mind does determine a lot about how you feel about yourself and who you become.

Self-talk is not just random thoughts and chatter in your mind. It creates its own reality. If you keep telling yourself that you can do something then it probably will happen. If you keep telling yourself that you can't accomplish something then you probably won't. How you see and relate to yourself is determined by your self-talk. It also may determine how others see you or how you present yourself in other people's eyes.

Your self-esteem and confidence is greatly impacted by your self-talk. Both positive and negative self-talk have a huge influence on how you feel. It is this negative self-talk that will cause the most damage. We are all our own worst critics and we just love to push the replay button and replay the negative events or shortcomings over and over. As you know, the more attention you give to those negative thoughts the harder it is to put them behind you.

Happy people seem to be able to put those occasional bad days behind them. According to a survey of 231 college students, all those with an overall positive outlook were the ones who were more likely to look back on a negative event and realize how much better things are for them today.

Depression is the outcome, unless you can get control of most of your negative self-talk. Yes, you can talk yourself in a serious case of depression, anxiety or other mood disorders. Research has found that those who have clinical depression have frequent and persistent destructive self-talk.

It can be difficult to turn 'Off' the negative self-talk. To do so you must have a plan or a simple system. Here are a few tips on how to turn off the negative self-talk.

- *Distance Yourself.* Even the strongest individual can't expel negative talk forever. You can however step back away from it for a bit.

- *Distract Yourself.* Try doing an activity that will fully engage your mind like a crossword puzzle, playing basketball, or working on your hobby.

- *Save Those Thoughts For Later*. Set some time aside later in the day for this negative conversation with yourself. When that time comes you might find that those negative thoughts have run out of steam.

- *Reprimand Them.* Your negative thoughts could just dissolve when you reprimand them.

Here are some tips on how to turn 'On' the positive self-talk. Just like trying to turn off the negative you must have a plan to turn on the positive talk.

- *Pay Attention To Your Self-talk.* Paying attention and listening to what you are saying to yourself will help you realize when you need to change the direction of your conversation.

- *Practice Positive Self-talk.* Like everything else in life, if you want to become good at something you have to practice.

- *Have Positive Thoughts In Reserve.* Have a few positive thoughts or statements ready to use when you catch yourself having a negative self-talk session. Just keep repeating these positive statements until the negative side of your conversation stops.

For good health, both physically and mentally you must eventually master the art of positive self-talk. You can master the skill by learning more about self-talk and then practice positive self-talk every day. Your body, mind and spirit will love you for it.

Action Item: Pay more attention to your self-talk and take appropriate action when you catch negative comments.

2. AS A MAN THINKETH

"For As A Man Thinketh In His Heart, So Is He." Proverbs 23:7

This simple idea is one of the most powerful concepts known to man, but is not fully understood nor practiced by many. It is all encompassing in your life. It literally dictates what transpires in your life. Control your thoughts and you control your circumstances, successes and your entire life.

An English gentleman by the name of James Allen wrote a book, **"As A Man Thinketh,"** that was published in 1901. He understood the importance of and the influence that your thoughts have on your personal life.

Here are a few thoughts from his book:

"A man is literally *what he thinks*, his character being the complete sum of all his thoughts."

"Man is made or unmade by himself; in the armory of thought he forges the weapons by which he destroys himself; he also fashions the tools with which he builds for himself heavenly mansions of joy and strength and peace."

"Every thought-seed sown or allowed to fall into the mind, and to take root there, produces its own, blossoming sooner or later into act, and bearing its own fruitage of opportunity and circumstances. Good thoughts bear good fruit, bad thoughts bad fruit."

"Not what he wishes and prays for does a man get, but what he justly earns. His wishes and prayers are only gratified and answered when they harmonize with his thoughts and actions."

"Disease and health, like circumstances, are rooted in thought."

"Until thought is linked with purpose there is no intelligent accomplishment."

"As the physically weak man can make himself strong by careful and patient training, so the man of weak thoughts can make them strong by exercising himself in right thoughts."

"A man can only rise, conquer, and achieve by lifting up his thoughts."

"Dream lofty dreams, and as you dream, so shall you become."

As you can see James Allen was a very thoughtful and insightful individual that has provided you and I with some serious things to think about. Change Your Thoughts – Change Your Life!

Action item: Read and Study "As A Man Thinketh" by James Allen   Reading time is about an hour or so. It will be a life changing experience.

3. AFFIRMATIONS - Reprogramming The Mind

af·firm·a·tion   ˌafərˈmāSH(ə)n/   *Noun*

1. The action or process of affirming something or being affirmed.
   Synonyms: declaration, statement, proclamation, pronouncement

2. Emotional support or encouragement.

From time to time we all have a problem with negative self-talk. Since this is true, you need to implement methods to help reprogram your mind towards positive self-talk.

Affirmations are one simple way to help reprogram your thoughts and provide yourself emotional support and encouragement.

Affirmations are generally short, concise, powerful and especially positive statements. These statements describe a desired goal or situation, and the statement is repeated often until it is imbedded into the subconscious mind.

When the statement(s) are repeated over and over the subconscious mind starts to work on your behalf to make the positive statement become a reality. Your subconscious mind will accept as the truth or reality whatever you keep saying to yourself or out loud. It will attract events or situations into your life that will help your statements come true. So it is important that only positive statements be used in affirmations in order to get positive results.

Tips on how to write and do affirmations:

1. Keep the affirmations short and not too long.
2. Use positive words with no negative undertones or references. Use a statement like "I am losing weight" instead of "I am not fat". Which statement brings positive images to your mind? The words you use have to bring a positive mental image of what you want.
3. Write the statements using the present tense such as, "I am totally relaxed and stress free", instead of "I will be totally relaxed and stress free". Can you feel and see the difference? The subconscious mind will work overtime to make a present statement happen now.
4. REPEAT these statements as often as possible throughout the day. Do not affirm while driving or any other activity that requires your full attention. You can try to set 5-10 minutes aside for special affirmation sessions several times a day. Repeat out loud when you are alone. Read them, think about them, and visualize the statements.
5. RELAX as much as possible when going over your affirmations. A relaxed body helps relax the mind.
6. FOCUS your full attention on each of the words that make up your affirmation.
7. FAITH in what you are sayings and having a strong Desire will bring faster results.
8. SEE and FEEL what you want to be true in your life. Then regardless of your current situation your subconscious mind will attract your affirmation into your life.

Here are some examples that you can use just the way they are, or you can modify them to match your personal desires.

Simple Affirmations:

- ♥ I have a lot of energy.
- ♥ My body is healthy and functioning in a very good way.
- ♥ I am calm and relaxed in every situation.
- ♥ I study and comprehend fast.
- ♥ I am living in the house of my dreams.
- ♥ I radiate love and happiness.
- ♥ My thoughts are under my control.
- ♥ I have a good and loving relationship with my wife/husband/child.
- ♥ I am successful in whatever I do.
- ♥ I have a wonderful and satisfying job.
- ♥ Everything is getting better and better every day.

More Complex Affirmations

- ➤ My thoughts are filled with positivity and my life is plentiful with prosperity.
- ➤ My efforts are being supported by the universe; my dreams manifest into reality before my eyes.
- ➤ My obstacles are moving out of my way; my path is pointed toward greatness.
- ➤ I am at peace with all that has happened, is happening now, and that will happen.
- ➤ I forgive those who have harmed me in my past and peacefully remove them and move on.
- ➤ Happiness is a choice. I base my happiness on my own accomplishments and the blessings I have been given.

Action item: Find or write 2 affirmations. Review and repeat these affirmations multiple times a day for 1 week.

4. THE PETER PAN SOLUTION - Happy Thoughts

Remember back a few years ago, the movie - 'HOOK'? This movie is about Peter Pan (played by Robin Williams) as an adult. He forgets that he is THE Peter Pan. Captain Hook kidnaps Peter Pans children and takes them back to 'Never Never Land' to make them pirates. Peter Pan had forgotten how to fly because he was an adult and forgotten about Never, Never Land.

In order to fight Captain Hook and to rescue his children from the pirates, Peter had to learn how to fly again. Tinker Bell knew the secret and told Peter Pan that he could not fly until he found and thought about his **"HAPPY THOUGHT"**. Once he found and thought about his happy thought Peter Pan could fly. For Peter it was the birth of his first child, his son.

You need to find **YOUR** – 'Happy Thought'. Your happy thought(s) can be about anything you want. The best happy thoughts are from an experience you had sometime in your life.

Think about this experience now. Try to remember how it felt. Remember the smells, the touch, the sounds, the taste and the feelings in your heart. Make the thought as real as possible. Try to re-live the moment.

How did that make you feel? Did this experience put a smile on your face? Did the current feelings of sadness or worry start to diminish?

Once you really get your Peter Pan Happy Thought down, use it daily when thoughts of sadness or worry start to plague your mind and watch those negative feeling melt away upon the arrival of your happy thought.

Action item: Remember and develop 2-3 "Happy Thoughts" and file them away in your mind for use on those sad or worry days.

RELATIONSHIPS

5. THE GOLDEN RULE - How To Treat People, Including Yourself

"Do unto others as you would have them do unto you."
Bible

This is the most familiar version of this thought.

This rule seems like a common sense way to live, but look around you. There are daily examples in the news where people are NOT treating others the way they would like to be treated. Some of these people seem to believe the opposite is the better way to live – 'Do unto others <u>before</u> they do it unto you.' So they will scam you, steal from you and maybe hurt you, before someone does it to them. This is a sad way to live life.

This idea, to treat others the way you would like them to treat you, is not just a Christian based rule. Similar rules can be found in most all religions, for example;

Buddhism   *Hurt not others in ways that you yourself would find hurtful.*
Udana-Varga 5,1

Hinduism   *This is the sum of duty; do naught onto others what you would not have them do unto you.*
Mahabharata 5,1517

Islam	*No one of you is a believer until he desires for his brother that which he desires for himself.* Sunnah
Judaism	*What is hateful to you, do not do to your fellowman. This is the entire Law; all the rest is commentary.* Talmud, Shabbat 3rd
Taoism	*Regard your neighbor's gain as your gain, and your neighbor's loss as your own loss.* Tai Shang Kan Yin P'ien

As you can see they all teach essentially the same principle. As you put this idea into practice, you will also find that others will treat you better.

Now here is a new twist to this idea. The golden rule applies to you and how you should treat yourself.

"Treat yourself the way you would want others to treat you."

Not everyone is going to treat you well, so at the very minimum you need to treat yourself well. Sometimes that is hard to do. It seems easy to treat others well while neglecting or even being hurtful to yourself. It takes a concerted effort to make sure your needs are being met while treating others well.

You are special so treat yourself special while you are treating everyone else special. Then watch most everyone else start treating you special in return. It works.

Action item: This week treat yourself with the Golden Rule and treat yourself like you would like others to treat you.

6.   HUGS - Give Them Away Daily

Who does not like a nice, warm, heart-felt hug? Very few people! Most of us love giving and receiving hugs from loved ones.

Hug Therapy is a great way of going through mental or physical healing. Research shows that hugging is effective and efficient at healing or reducing depression, anxiety, stress and loneliness. It is also great at healing sickness and diseases.

Hugs are the next step up from a handshake. When you hold out your hand, this is an invitation to shake hands. When it comes to hugs I always suggest that you ask permission first. This is especially important if it is not a close friend or family member. Many people are not use to being hugged, so ask first, and then hug.

The type of hug I am talking about is a proper deep hug; one where the hearts are pressing together. Some people call this a 'Bear Hug'. Research is showing that this type of hug has the following benefits:

1. First and foremost, the nurturing and loving touch of a hug helps build a sense of safety and trust. A hug helps you to have an open and honest communication with others.

2. Increases your Oxytocin levels almost instantly. Oxytocin helps heal feelings of anger, loneliness and isolation.
3. Hugs help teach you that love flows both ways. Hugs also teach us how to give and receive. There is equal value in giving and receiving.

4. Hugs are a lot like laughter and meditation. You are taught to let go and be present in the moment. Hugs let you get

out of your mundane and circular thinking patterns so you can connect with your heart, your feelings and your breath. Hugs allow you to flow the energy of life.

5. Serotonin levels are increased when we hold a hug for more than a brief second. Your moods will elevate and help create more happiness. Let your hugs linger just a bit longer.

6. Your self-esteem gets a nice boost from hugging. Since you were a baby the touch from your family shows you that you are special and loved. There is an association between self-worth and physical sensations from your earliest years and that is still imbedded in your nervous system today. All those cuddles you received from your parents while growing up still remain imprinted at a cellular level. Hugs remind us at a somatic level of those cuddling moments; therefore, hugs connect you to your ability to self-love.

7. Your muscles relax and tension is released from your body when you hug. Pain dissipates for a little while after a hug.

8. There is an energy that is exchanged between two people when they are hugging. This is an investment in that relationship. Hugs encourage understanding and empathy. There is a synergistic effect, which means that 'the whole is greater than the sum of its parts'. This synergy can cause a win-win-win outcome – you, the other person and the relationship all wiin.

9. Hugs help balance the nervous system. There is a galvanic skin response with the person giving and receiving a hug, which shows a change in the skin conductance. The effect in the moisture and electricity in the skin suggests that the

parasympathetic nervous system is in a more balanced state.

10. Your immune system is strengthened by hugs. The gentle pressure on your sternum and the emotional charge that is created activates the Solar Plexus Chakra. This helps stimulate your thymus gland (this regulates and balances your body's production of white blood cell, which keep you healthy and disease free).

Based on these 10 benefits, you can see that there are a lot of benefits from receiving and giving hugs.

Hugs improve relationships and elevate moods, so set a goal for 10-12 hugs a day. 4-5 hugs a day will do, but the bare minimum is 1 hug a day. To make this more of a challenge, give these hugs to different people and not just the same individuals each time. It will brighten your day and the other person's day.

Virginia Satir, is a highly respected family therapist and she had this to say about hugs.

"We need four hugs a day for survival. We need eight hugs a day for maintenance. We need twelve hugs a day for growth."

Action Item: Give away at least 2 hugs every day, and then work up from there. Remember to ask permission first.

7. TOUCH - Humans Thrive On Physical Touch

There is nothing more emotionally and physically healing than human touch. When we touch each other, there is a spiritual connection and an exchange of energy that is recognized at the subconscious level.

Humans need to feel physical touch. You have a deep need to be touched and also to touch others. They in return want and need to be touched. We are talking appropriate touching, such as a hug (with permission), shaking hands, holding hands, lightly placing a hand on a shoulder or arm.

I have done a lot of work with the elderly through a service assignment in my church and I always shake their hands, hold their hands or lightly place my hand on their hands or arms when talking to them. I feel their love and they feel mine. We both benefit from this slight touch.

Research seems to back this all up!

At Duke University in North Carolina, research is showing that touch and massage can cut down on the levels of stress hormones. These elevated stress hormones are responsible for increasing your risk of a number of diseases and mood disorders. Touch seems to increase the levels of melatonin and serotonin.

The Touch Research Institute at the University Of Miami School Of Medicine says that they hav performed more than 100 studies into human touch and found it has significant effects on the following:

- Faster growth in premature babies

- Reduced Pain
- Lower glucose levels in children with diabetes
- Improved immune system in people with cancer
- Decrease autoimmune disease symptoms.

As you can see, human touch has healing properties. You never know who might need a 'healing touch'. Touch spreads love, and love heals everything, so spread love wherever you go. Others will feel better and you will feel better.

ACTION ITEM: Start touching people in a natural, non-invasive way to let them know you care. Touch transmits love, and love heals everything.

8. LISTEN - Listen Twice As Much As You Talk

The title of this tip is a correct principle BUT when you are listening really listen. You have to not only hear what is being said, but more importantly you must understand what they are saying.

Listening skills is one of the most important talent you can have. How well you listen has a major impact on your job effectiveness, and on the quality of your relationships with others.

There are 4 major reasons why we listen. We listen –

- To obtain information.
- To Understand
- For Enjoyment.
- To Learn.

Improved listening skills will help you at work and at home. Much of the stress in life comes from misunderstandings, either at work with co-workers or at home with family members. Most of the misunderstanding comes from not 'listening' to the other person. Yes, you may 'hear' them but did you listen to them and get all the information that they were trying to pass on to you.

Here are a couple of listening tips.

1. PAY ATTENTION - Give the speaker your undivided attention, and acknowledge the message.
2. SHOW THAT YOU ARE LISTENING - Use your own body language and gestures to convey your attention.
3. PROVIDE FEED BACK - As a listener, your role is to understand what is being said. This may require you to reflect what is being said and ask questions.
4. DO NOT INTERUPT or DEFER JUDGMENT - Interrupting is a waste of time. It frustrates the speaker and limits full understanding of the message.
5. APPROPRIATELY RESPOND - You are gaining information and perspective. You add nothing by attacking the speaker or otherwise putting him or her down.

If you will improve your listening skill and really listen to the one who is speaking, and listen twice as much as you talk, the relationships will improve. This improved relationship and improved effectiveness at work will also help reduce stress. We know that stress leads to sickness, disease and depression.

So for your health and your happiness, LISTEN!!

ACTION ITEM: When someone is talking, implement these 5 tips. Listen and stop thinking about YOUR next response back. Remember – when the other person is talking, what they are saying is the most important thing going on at that moment.

9. FORGIVE OTHERS AND YOURSELF - Then Let It Go

> **Forgiveness** – *The decision and act of letting go of and to stop feeling, angry, resentment and thoughts of revenge.*

The act of forgiveness can and will lessen the grip that someone, who has offended or hurt you, may have on you. It will help you focus on other more positive parts of your life. When you forgive someone you do not necessarily forget the wrong that was done, but it can and will lead to feelings of empathy, compassion and understanding for the one who hurt you.

The Attitude of forgiving and forgiveness helps release stress that may be bottled up inside of you. Forgiveness is another great stress reliever.

This need to forgive is not just for the big things someone has done to you but also the little things, such as someone cutting you off on the freeway, a mean comment or a rude act. You don't even have to forgive them in person. If someone cuts you off on the freeway, you just think to yourself (or you can say it out loud), 'you must have a good reason so I forgive you', then let it go.

There are two sides of the forgiveness coin. The other side of this forgiveness step is for YOU to apologize and ask for forgiveness, to all those that you may have offended. None of us is perfect and this includes you. Take responsibility for your words and actions and when you offend someone – apologize.

But here is the catch. You must feel truly sorry for whatever you have said or done. You must be sincere in your sorrow or regret and specifically, <u>you need to ask for forgiveness and do it without making any excuses.</u>

Remember one thing, the other person may or may not accept your apology and forgive you. You cannot force them to forgive you. It may take them time to be moved enough to forgive. What is important is that you <u>sincerely</u> apologize.

Now that you have apologized to the person that you may have treated badly, you must now forgive yourself! This is the hardest step for most people. You are your own worst critic. You should not judge yourself too harshly. You are human, and as such you will make mistakes.

Very often depression is the result of excessive self-criticism that takes place over an extended period of time. These self-criticisms are sometimes the result of guilty feelings, plus it is easy to go overboard on beating yourself up.

I can almost promise that as you let go of grudges and bad feelings towards another person and yourself, you will no longer let your life be defined by how you have been hurt. You stop being the victim. You might be lucky enough to find understanding and compassion.

So forgive others, apologize and forgive yourself, quickly.

ACTION ITEM: Forgive someone every day, including YOU. Apologize when necessary. Never carry guilt or anger in your heart for long.

10. EAT MEALS TOGETHER AS A FAMILY

Eating together as a family could also mean with friends, as couples or extended family. You can even count eating lunch with co-workers if you are single. But for most of you it would be with loved ones.

You are probably wondering why eating together is so important. Well, most American families do not eat many meals together. Families are lacking in face time together and even having meaningful conversations with each other. Dinner may be the only time during the day that you can sit down to eat and have a conversation as a family.

Dinner should be a time where family can come together to relax, laugh, recharge their physical and emotional batteries. You can catch up on the activities of all the family members. This is a great time to build a sense of who your family is and develop closeness to each other. Mealtime creates a feeling of togetherness and family cohesion.

I know that your family is probably extremely busy but if your family could eat 5 meals a week together, your family and you personally will receive some great benefits. Researchers have found the following benefits for eating at least 5 meals a week together.

- Builds a healthy body and brain
- Great for building family spirit
- Lower Teenage substance abuse and pregnancy
- Lower Depression rates in teenagers
- Increased self-esteem and grades in children and teens
- Diet is greatly improved – improved health condition

- Less Obesity and other eating disorders
- Conversation is better at building vocabulary than reading

There are also a few other benefits for parents and adults.

- Your moods are elevated and there is less depression and anxiety
- Children will stay closer to you as parents than those children who do not eat with their parents
- For couples without children, you become closer or stay closer to your spouse, because of conversation
- Eating together around the dinner table can be a great 'unifier', a place all family members can feel safe.

One last point – eating alone can feel very lonely and alienating. This can help foster depression, anxiety and other mood disorders. So if you are depressed, feeling down or upset with a family member, sitting down and eating with them or others helps heal the wounds of loneliness or anger.

"A Family That Eats Together Stays Together And All Members Are Healthier and Happier."

ACTION ITEM: Eat Dinner together as a family, around the table, today. Try for 5 or more home cooked Dinners (or other meals) a week as a family. Your body, mind, spirit and family will love you for it.

11. FRIENDSHIP - Quality Not Quantity

The research is in and shows that if you have a strong social network of good, strong, positive and committed friends you have a significant increase in better health and living longer. The reverse is also true – if you are socially isolated, you have a higher risk of poor mental and physical health and a shorter lifespan.

The research also shows that a few good friends that have a positive outlook on life and are usually in a good mood can have a far greater positive impact on the rest of the group. This is especially true if one within the group is suffering from depression or illness. Having a small group of dedicated friends can help you heal faster from illness, surgery or a mood disorder.

Here is one more thing to think about concerning friends. Acquaintances are NOT Friends. Casual friends or acquaintances probably will not be there for you in time of physical or emotional hardships. Real friends will!

"To Get A Friend - You Have To Be A Friend"

Here is story about how to be a friend – A story of a young man's SMILE during his hardship.

Jaden Hayes, a six year old boy, whose parents had both died, was understandably heartbroken. Even though his parents were gone, he was determined to go on living with joy and happiness. One day he told his aunt that he was 'sick and tired of seeing everyone so sad all the time.'

So he decided he wanted to help turn other people's frowns into smiles. So Jaden, at the age of 6, started a 'Smile Campaign'. So

Jaden and his aunt started handing out toys. These toys were small rubber duckies, dinosaurs, etc. – in order to make people, who were not smiling, Smile. His goal was 33,000 people smiling. At the time of the story he had made about 500 people smile.

Jaden is proof that even if you are going through a tough time, you can still make a difference in someone else's life, helping both of you heal. Smile often to others, even strangers, and you will feel better and so will the other person. Who knows, maybe that smile will be the start of another great friendship.

ACTION ITEMS: Using some of the previous tips do something today to strengthen the relationship with a close, dear friend. You might really need them someday. Smile and Say Hi to a stranger today and brighten both your days.

12. SPOUSES – Give and Receive Love and Intimacy

There are many studies that show that if you are in a loving relationship you have a much lower death rate compared to a single person. If you are in a strong, supportive and healthy relationship you will have a higher level of self-esteem which means you will be less likely developing depression. Also, a loving relationship will help you reduce anxiety levels.

Research also tells us, along with common sense and experience, that couples who are having sexual intimacy on a regular basis have longer lasting marriages. These couples report that they are healthier and overall happier.

43

Intimacy, including sexual contact, is very important to your health and wellbeing. Every type of physical intimacy such as holding hands, kissing, and hugging is a nonverbal way of showing your spouse that you care for them and that you find them attractive. You also communicate to them that they are desired, cherished and very important in the relationship.

Here are some tips on improving your relationships by giving and receiving love and intimacy.

- Cuddle more. Snuggling up into each other's arms while watch TV or a movie will help release some of those 'feel good' hormones.

- Hug and kiss your spouse at least 3 times every day. Once on the way to work, when you return home from work and just before going to bed.
  - Kissing for good health
    - Burns calories: It may only be 6 calories a minute but what a fun way to burn those calories!
    - Relieves Stress: Cortisol levels drop while kissing, a sign that you are relaxing.
    - Healthier Teeth: Kissing activates your saliva glands which actually washes off harmful bacteria and reduces plaque buildup.

- Hold hands, even in public. Hold hands on walks, shopping and yes, even attending church services.

- Massage each other's neck and shoulders. We all know that even simple massages can be very relaxing, therapeutic and great for maintaining good health.

It really is more about touching each other than anything else. It is these simple acts of physical intimacy that can bring you the most healing and improvement to your health and relationship.

One last word on this! Don't wait for your spouse to lead out on this. This works both ways – In The Giving and In The Receiving. Reciprocation is the key! Enjoy!

ACTION ITEM: Talk to your spouse and find 1 area of intimacy that you will both improve on.

Example – Implement the 3 hugs/kisses a day!

13.   THE INNER LOVE: SELF-LOVE

"Before you can truly love someone else you must first love yourself." Do you believe this statement to be true? There are many variations to this statement, but they are all true. The fact is, you must love yourself before you can really love someone else.

Here is another one that I recently read, *"Your relationship with others is a mirror of your relationship with yourself."* In other words, if you have 'less than desirable' relationship with a loved one, please take a good hard look inside. The problem could be the relationship you have with yourself. Take care of the relationship you have with yourself and the problems you may have with others just may disappear.

I know you like the good feelings you get when you do things for others. But doing things for others really does not bring you lasting happiness. What is more important is how you see or perceive yourself for doing the good things for others, which really determine whether you are really feeling 'happy'.

There is a difference between the two. It is a good thing to help others but it is the reason or motivation behind it that really counts. Consider this for a moment. Are you helping others just because you need to feel good about yourself? Do you need other people's feedback to feel good about yourself? If so, it is because you have a limited ability to feel good about yourself without this positive feedback! Or in other words – You Lack Self-Love!

What if you had more self-love and self-acceptance? If so, all the positive feedback and responses that you may get when you help someone would not be so important to you. Once you have found and develop love and acceptance for you, then the reason to help others changes from a form of self-gratification or self-love to doing it out of love for them and yourself.

Who you are, your true self, your inner goodness is found within your inner core or your divine nature. You do not have to be different to be worthy of your own love. Because of your divine nature you are love. You are a wonderful and beautiful light. Believe in yourself and let your love and light shine forth and do not try to bury that love and light.

Loving yourself is a journey, an ongoing process and even a lifetime pursuit – and it all starts with YOU. So give yourself a great big hug and a few words of encouragement and try some of the following tips.

- o Stop comparing yourself to others! You are a special and unique individual. There is nobody like you. So only compare yourself with the only person looking back at you in the mirror. Be kind and gentle with that person.

- When you wake up every morning, look in the mirror and tell yourself something really positive. It can be an affirmation, positive feedback on how you handled a situation, just something positive and something that will make you smile.
- When you are having a fantastic day, sit down and write out a list of your best qualities and accomplishments. Then on those days that are less than amazing, pull out the list and read it.

Be patient but be persistent. Self-Love is process and sometimes it can be a slow process, but keep taking steps forward. It takes daily practice and a life time to master but it can and must be mastered.

So be kind to yourself. Support yourself especially when facing hard times.

ACTION ITEM: Every morning give yourself a big hug and tell yourself something positive and that will make you smile. Remember – You have to love yourself before you can truly love someone else.

CAREER

14. RELATIONSHIP WITH MONEY

Did you know that your relationship with money started when you were a child? Your attitude about money is generally passed down from your parents. This subconscious belief system about money is called Money Scripts. It is these Money Scripts that drive your financial behaviors and decisions.

Having a poor relationship with money can be a major cause of stress in your life. Stress leads to mental and physical diseases. You must have a good, positive and strong relationship with money to reduce stress and maintain a healthy and happy life.

Signs of a good relationship with money may include:

- No or low debt
- Spending money based on your values, needs and based on priorities
- Having and sticking to a budget
- Having an emergency fund and insurance
- Saving money in order to meet your goals and obtaining wants
- An attitude that money is not evil and can be used for good.

If you have a lot of debt, spend money on impulse, have no budget or emergency funds and have a bad attitude about money, then you really need to work on your relationship with money.

Here are a couple of ideas to get you started.

❖ Attitude – It is all about Attitude. First be very thankful for everything you <u>do have</u> and worry less about what you <u>don't have</u>.

❖ WANTS and NEEDS – There is a difference. NEEDS are things like basic food, shelter, clothing, transportation and a job. WANTS are things like a large screen TV, sports car, eating at fancy restaurants, and wearing all the latest top fashion name brand clothes. You must know and understand the difference between NEEDS and WANTS.

Life will go a little smoother, with less stress and with more happiness, when you have a great relationship with money.

Action Item: List your needs and wants. Then prioritize the wants. Try setting aside a little money each month towards the purchase of the #1 item on your 'Wants' List.

15. STRESS CONTRIBUTOR - Your Job

"Chronic job strain can put both your physical and emotional health at risk."
Paul J. Rosch MD   American Institute of Stress

As you may well know, your job can be one of the major contributors to your higher levels of stress. You may also be aware of the fact that chronic stress is the leading cause of sickness, disease and mood disorders like depression and anxiety.

You may also feel like you have no control over the stress associated with your job. But there is a lot you can do about it. The first step is determining what part(s) of your job are contributing to your stress. Once you know the causes, or what triggers the stress, you can then start to lay out a plan to try to reduce those triggers.

You spend as many hours at work as you do at home with your family and loved ones. It should be as stress free as possible. Find ways to reduce the stress at work and you will find more peace, happiness and health in your life.

Tips 16-21, once implemented into your life will almost assure your work related stress levels will be down to a minimum. These tips will help you reduce your work related stress. Maybe it is because you are not "working your dream job".

ACTION ITEM: Evaluate your job or career and list the areas of your job that cause you the most stress. Mark those items that you may have some control over and then list things you can change that will help reduce the work stress.

16. LEARN TO LOVE THE JOB

Yes, it is possible to learn to love your current job. For your health and sanity you must learn to love your current job or learn how to tolerate the job until you can find a job that you can love. I want you to read and really think about this next comment. You may not like nor agree with it but think about it and see if it might just apply to you.

"People Change Jobs Because They Will Not Change Themselves."

Some experts agree with this statement and have said that sometimes YOU are the one who needs to change, not the job. It really does not matter what is causing your bad outlook or attitude about your job. You need to take a look at all the different aspects of your job and figure out what you can change and what you cannot change. Then work on those items that you can change.

"YOUR JOB DOES NOT DEFINE YOU, BUT HOW YOU DO IT DOES."

The real trick is to take control and don't let the job define who you are. What really counts is how you do your job and your attitude about your performance. Chances are you focus on the things you cannot control. Start looking at what you can control. Focus on the positive factors of your job and work on changing those things about your job that you can. As you do, you will start to see things differently about your job and you just might come to love the job you have.

- Learn as much as you can about your job. Ask to be crossed trained in several other areas. It will be a change of pace plus it will make you more valuable to the company.
- Bring treats to work for the co-workers. This will help lighten the mood and make for a less stressful day.

Your health and happiness depends on your satisfaction with your job or career. You can learn to love your job. It may be work but it will be well worth the investment.

ACTION ITEM: Memorize this statement and try to put it into practice at work each day. It will help you enjoy your job more.

"There are times when you can't control your situation, but you can always choose how you live in it."

17.   ARE YOU WORKING YOUR DREAM?   It Is Not Too Late!

Ask yourself these questions –

- Am I working the job / career of my dreams?
- If I knew I could not fail, what would I do today to support my family?
- If I could turn back the clock, what career decision would I change?

Because you spend so much of your life at work you must be relatively happy while you are there. Most people and I suspect even you are not working your dream job or working in your dream career. Why not? One of the biggest reasons is because of fear!

You were afraid to go to school because you were not smart enough, or now you think you are too old to go back to school. Maybe you are afraid that you would fail at business, or that you may actually be successful. We all have reasons for not working our dreams.

It is not too late to change. No matter what anyone else tells you, 'IT IS NEVER TOO LATE TO CHANGE DIRECTIONS AND GET ON ANOTHER CAREER PATH'!

It is vitally important to have a job or career that you can get very excited and motivated about. It needs to get you into bed early with anticipation of a new day and cause you to bounce out of bed in the morning when the alarm goes off. This kind of job/career will be a huge boost to your health and happiness.

ACTION ITEM: Answer this question – What would you be doing right now, IF you knew you would be successful?

Once you have the answer nailed down go to work to make it a reality.

18. ENTREPRENEURSHIP - Is It For You

Have you ever dreamed of owning your own business, being your own boss? Many entrepreneurs absolutely love what they are doing. Do they say it is easy and a piece of cake? No. They will all tell you that it can be stressful, a lot of work, and even discouraging at times. But they will quickly tell you that it is worth it.

Is going into business right for you? Well that all depends. Starting a business does not have to be complicated but it does take a little money, time and a whole lot of commitment and perseverance. But you can do it.

Here is a list of healthy reasons to start your own business.

- Many entrepreneurs are healthier than the average wage earner.

- On average, business owners eat healthier than non-business owners.
- They exercise more, up to 30 minutes 3-5 times a week.
- Entrepreneurs are more optimistic about the future.
- Once the business is established they have more free time to enjoy life.

Researchers are starting to discover that entrepreneurs live longer and are healthier than employees. There are a variety of reasons for this. Here is one such study found in The Journal of Occupational and Organizational Psychology.

Here the researchers compared the health of a nationally representative sample of employees and entrepreneurs and then they examined a wide range of health factors from both these groups. These health factors include areas such as mental illness, physical disease, and sick days taken, number of visits to the doctor, and their overall well-being and their satisfaction with their lives.

The results? Entrepreneurs were the healthiest group in essentially every area. These individuals had much lower rates of mental illnesses such as depression and anxiety (the two leading mental health issues in the world today), less physical illnesses such as high blood pressure, hypertension, lower rates of hospital visits and they just felt better all the way around.

As you can see, entrepreneurship has some very positive, healthy advantages. But again you have to be doing something that you love doing and providing a product or service that you are passionate about. It will be worth your time to research what it will take to start a business in an area that you love. You never know, you might become a very successful business owner.

ACTION ITEM:** Read a book about how to start and run your own business. See if you have the passion, determination and personality to be an entrepreneur.* ***OR *List subjects that you are passionate about and have expertise in. Then research business ideas that are within that subject area.*

19.   FIND THE WORK YOU LOVE

2,500 years ago Aristotle gave us one of the best career advices ever given –

"Where the needs of the world and your talents cross, there lies your vocation."

Recent research has shown that those individuals who pursue money and status are less likely to feel fulfillment in their career. Aristotle would agree with these researchers. In addition Harvard University professor Howard Gardner said, 'The best alternative is to find an ethical career, focused on values and issues that matter to YOU, and which also allows you to do what you're really good at.'

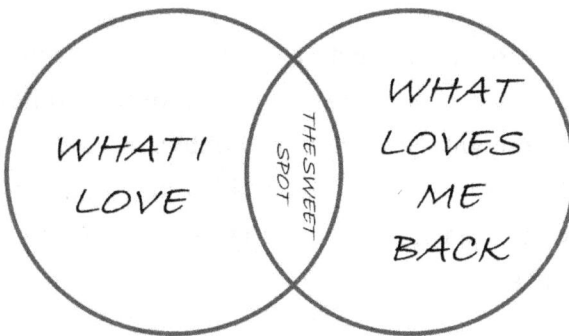

WHAT I LOVE

THE SWEET SPOT

WHAT LOVES ME BACK

Here is a way to find this special 'zone' that you need to be in. Get a paper and pen. Draw a circle on the paper just off to the left a little. Now to the right just a little, draw another circle and overlap the other circle just a bit. This will create three areas or zones. Label the left circle 'What I Love' and in the right circle write 'What Loves You Back'. The left circle represents your passions or skill sets that you love to do. The right circle represents jobs or careers that give back to you in such things as pay and satisfaction. Now look at the zone in the middle. That is where you want to be. Doing what you love AND getting pay and satisfaction for doing it.

What is stopping you from entering the 'zone'? For most people it is FEAR. If you ask all those who have successfully changed careers, how to overcome this fear they will probably tell you the same thing. 'STOP THINKING ABOUT IT AND JUST DO IT!' You have to take a chance.

This may be why most all cultures through-out history have come to realize that if you want to have and live a meaningful, abundant and vibrant life, you have to take some chances. If not, you might end up having a life full of regrets. This is not what you want. So take a calculated risk.

One way to do it is to start out with a day job, that you may not like, that covers your bills, while you test out other options on the side. You can experiment with your ideas or hobbies but give the ideas time to develop. If after a while you decide that you do not like doing that particular idea as much as you thought, you can move on to something else.

You don't have to take huge risks when you 'take a chance' on a different career path. Here are a couple of questions to ask yourself to get ideas on what you might like to try.

'What is one thing I have gotten the most enjoyment from throughout my life? Why?'

'IF money (pay check) was not an issue, what would I do every day?'

'What job or career would I be excited to tell everyone about?'

These are just a few that you could ask yourself and ponder over for a while. The important thing to remember is, your life will be freer from stress and you will find more happiness and fulfillment in life if you are working at a job or in a career that you love. It will be worth the effort to find this somewhat allusive dream.

ACTION ITEM: Draw out the circle diagram and list all the things you love to do, what those things will give you back and see if you can find a realistic, workable zone in the middle.

20.   PASSIONS AND HOBBIES

For many people and this may include you, would love to turn a passion or a hobby into a business or a source of income. This would be an ideal situation for finding a job that you could love. Let's take a minute and find out the difference between a *passion* and a *hobby* and see which one might be the one to pursue.

HOBBY – is a pursuit or activity that is outside of your regular occupation that is engaged in for relaxation. If you are doing something you enjoy, but not many people are willing to pay for doing it, this is a hobby and not a sustainable career.

With a hobby there are two different approaches – you will either need to work hard, learn more skills, knowledge or experience until people will pay you for it OR be content to keep it as a hobby purely for your enjoyment and relaxation.

PASSION – they don't leave you alone and are generally not relaxing. A Passion pushes itself in your life even if you don't have time for them. Passions will soothe you and at the same time can drive you crazy.

Passions are so much more than just a mere interest. They are a very strong interest and for some people, the passion almost takes over their lives. If you are passionate about something, you spend all or most of your free time on it. You are learning all you can and enhancing your skills in this area. You are always thinking about what you are going to do next with it.

With a passion, you are not afraid to work for it, and in fact you never consider IT work, but a pleasure to do. So, what are you willing to sacrifice time, money, sleep or a vacation for? What is the activity or area that you just can't stay away from? The answer would be your passion!

NOTE: There is a difference between Passion and Compulsion! You can control a passion, you can't control a compulsion. Know the difference. Compulsions control your life and are very negative. Passions and hobbies should be relaxing, refreshing, and pleasurable and can be turned into businesses and careers.

The whole idea behind this secret is that it is possible to develop a hobby, which then is turned into a passion. This new passion can then be turned into a career. Those who can do this will find more peace, fulfillment and happiness in their career. It is critical to your overall health and happiness to have a job or career that you love. Even if you feel that you cannot turn this hobby or passion into an income, you must have a hobby or something you can get passionate about just to make life a little more relaxing and enjoyable.

ACTION ITEM: Take a look at all your different activities and see which ones are hobbies or passions. Then evaluate to see if you can turn either into a source of income.

21. EDUCATION - The Road Away From Poverty

"Education is better than playing the lottery if you want to better your lifestyle."

We all seem to know that the more education you can get the better job you can qualify for. Research and statistics back up this idea.

- If you only have a high school education, you are ½ as likely to make over $40,000 a year compared to those with a college degree.

- If you have a college degree, you are nearly 9 times more likely to make over $100,000 a year and 13 times more likely to earn over $200,000 compared to someone with just a high school diploma

- By 2018 it is forecast that nearly 2/3 of all occupations in the U.S. will require a college degree.

A less expensive option is a two-year degree or trade certifications and many of these pay $50,000-$60,000 a years after a couple of years' experience. Check out your local community college and see what they have to offer.

Here is another option to consider – On the job training. Always keep an eye open for training opportunities at your current job. Learn all you can about your current job and then cross train in other areas.

NEVER STOP LEARNING! LEARNING IS A LIFETIME PERSUIT!

EDUCATION IS THE PATH TO A FINANCIALLY STABLE LIFE.

ACTION ITEM: Check into furthering your education. Check out the local community college, Online Universities and local colleges, no matter your age.

When it comes to education, the old wives tail – "You Can't Teach An Old Dog New Tricks" is false. You can do it!

PHYSICAL ACTIVITY (EXERCISE)

22.   30 MINUTES A DAY

Both webmd.com and the Mayo Clinic support the exercise recommendations of the U.S. Dept. of Health and Human Services. These are recommendations that will help maintain a good healthy body and mind. Their recommendations are minimums – more will be required for weight-loss:

- o Moderate Aerobic Activities – 30 minutes a day or 150 minutes a week. This type of activity would include – brisk walking, swimming, and mowing the lawn (riding lawn mowers do not count).
- o Vigorous Aerobic Exercise – 15 minutes a day or 75 minutes a week. This type of activity would include running or aerobic dancing.
- o Strength Training – Twice a week. There is no specific amount of time for each session. This type of activity would include weight machines or weight bearing exercises.

Here are three tips to help you implement 30 minutes of physical activities into your day:

1. Physical activities do not mean you have to "exercise". Make a list of physical activities you enjoy doing. Start doing some of these every day.
2. Involve others. Do these activities as a family or with a group of friends. This way all of you will benefit from the activity.
3. Start simple by taking the stairs, park farther away and walk, or take short walks around your office building.

Starting small and working up is simple to do and the health benefits are tremendous. Everyone knows exercise is good of you but few seem to put forth the effort. Your reward for adding more physical activities into your day life is great health and happiness. It is very hard to be happy when you feel tired and out of energy. Your body, mind and moods will love you for your efforts.

ACTION ITEM: Add more movement and physical activities into your daily routine. Strive for 30 total minutes a day of physical activities such as walking, taking the stairs or simple exercises.

23.   EXERCISE: VARIETY = SUSTAINABILITY

Variety is the spice of life when it comes to sticking to an exercise plan. Scientific studies support this idea. Many people start an exercise routine but quit after a few weeks. Now the prevailing wisdom is to add variation to your exercise routine to help keep you exercising. This is according to a University of Florida study.

This study was published in the Journal of Sport Behavior. The researchers took 114 men and women and put them into three categories or groups: Group 1 – exercise was varied. Group 2 – performed the same set of exercises and Group 3 – no set schedule or regulations.

Results: At the end of the study, there were only 61 of the 114 original members. 52 members had dropped out and one was disqualified. This left 24 people in the first group, 22 in the second group and only 15 in the third group. According to the researcher the highest dropout rate was with the 3rd group – with no schedule or regulations.

After the study researchers had the following tips and ideas;

- Do whatever it take to keep your routine from getting boring and monotonous
- Doing cardio exercises one day then the next day doing strength training and next day working on flexibility and alternating these three is the best routine for overall health, wellness and weight loss.
- If working out at home, walk one day, run the next and then aerobics. Just mix it up.
- Try new things. Try swimming, hiking, basketball… you get the idea.

Again, research proves that you will stick with exercising IF you make it fun, mix it up and involve others. In the end, it will be your willingness to try new things that will keep boredom away and increase your dedication to exercising… which will pay great dividends, including weight-loss, happier moods and overall better health.

ACTION ITEM: Mix it up by trying more new exercises, while keeping with those you found to be enjoyable. Your willingness to try new exercises or physical activities will lead to compliance and sustainability.

24. QI GONG - Movements For Health

The word Qigong (Chi Kung, Qigung) has two parts – Qi and Gong.

Qi is pronounced as 'Chee" which is translated to mean – *Life Force or Vital-Energy*. The Chinese believe this Life Force or Vital-Energy flows through all things in the universe.

Gong is pronounced as 'gung' and is translated to mean – **Skill or Accomplishment that is cultivated through steady practice**.

Qigong = Cultivating Life Force Energy

What is Qigong?

As an ancient Chinese health system, Qi gong integrates breathing techniques, physical movements and postures, and focused intentions. It has been practiced by the Chinese for centuries and goes back for several thousand years. Every day it is practiced by 10's of millions of people all around the world.

Qigong helps promote mental clarity, good health and has been shown to be effective in relieving a variety of ailments, including stress. Scientific research has shown that stress is a major contributing factor in depression, high blood pressure, asthma and heart disease, to list just a few issues. Because there is a lot of interest around the world in relieving stress, people are looking into the healing properties of Qigong. It is sometimes called **'moving meditation.'**

There are hundreds of variations of Qigong but all types of Qigong have the same three components:

- Postures – Movements
- Breathing techniques
- Mental Focus or Visualization

Most of the Qigong forms are slow and gentle movements that are easily adaptable and can even be done by the physically challenged and can be practiced by the old as well as the young. In China all ages, from the little children to the oldest sages, practice Qigong.

It is a system that is practiced to increase vitality and to promote healing and maintaining good health.

You will have a more positive outlook on life, and harmful attitudes, moods and behaviors will be eliminated, when the three characteristics of Qigong are unified and united. Incorporating Qigong into your daily routine will help create a well-balanced life style. When your life is more in balance it will bring greater harmony, stability and enjoyment into your daily life.

As you add the practice of Qigong into your daily life you will improve your physical health, mental health and your emotional health. In other words, you will improve your health and happiness in your life.

ACTION ITEM: Learn the Shibashi 18 Movements. Easy to learn and powerful, you will see great results.

25. YOGA - IF You Are Limber Enough

Yoga is to India as Qi Gong is to China. They use these different movements and poses to heal the mind and body in their respective countries.

Yoga is very popular and is practiced by athletes, children, seniors and people of all walks of life. Yoga can be modified to suit all levels of fitness, from beginners to the expert. It has been proven to lower blood pressure, increase flexibility and strength, and to reduce stress levels. Yoga calms the mind and energizes the body and mind.

So what exactly is Yoga? Most people picture people in weird, twisted and seemingly impossible poses. It is that and a lot more. Because of the poses many people feel they cannot do Yoga. I for one am not very flexible and have a nearly impossible time doing most of the poses. For this reason I stick with Qi Gong. But again Yoga is much more than the poses.

The word Yoga is derived from the Sankrit word "yuj" which means "to unite or integrate"; yoga is 5000 years old and originates from India. Yoga, for many people is a way of life, but for the rest of us it is way to relax, stretch and harmonize the body with the mind. Yoga does this through three main processes:

- Various Breathing Techniques (discussed in a later secret)
- Yoga Postures (your body needs to be pretty flexible to do many of these poses)
- Meditation (discussed in another secret)

66

When your body, mind and spirit are in harmony within you, your journey through life becomes a little calmer, happier and more fulfilled. There are many, many studies that show that Yoga helps heal so many different physical, mental and emotional issues that everyone can benefit from adding Yoga into their daily routine.

Here are some physical benefits of Yoga:

- Increased flexibility
- Improved muscle tone and strength
- Respiration, Vitality and Energy levels are improved
- A balanced metabolism and weight reduction
- Improved Circulatory and Cardio health

Beside these and many other physical benefits, one of the best or well-known benefits has to do with stress management. Stress as you may be well aware of, has a major impact on the body and mind. Stress is a major contributor to depression, anxiety, sleep disorders, and lack of concentration, just to list a few.

So to sum things up – "Yoga is effective in developing coping skills and reaching a more positive outlook on life."

Remember: Your body is your best guide. You don't have to stick to one kind of yoga, just do what your body needs, and try different types until you find one you like! Yoga can be one important step toward finding health and happiness. Try it! You just might like it!

ACTION ITEM: Find a local Yoga studio and register for a class or order a training video and try Yoga in the privacy of your own home. See if your body is flexible enough to do it.

26. THE BRAIN - It Needs Exercise Too

"If Your Brain Is Not Healthy And Happy – NOBODY Is Happy!"

Your brain is just like a muscle in your body. If you work it – it will grow and get stronger. If you do not use it – it will shrink and grow weaker. Many scientific studies prove this out. The growth of new brain cells and neurotransmitters is called neuroplasticity.

As you age or when there is repeated head trauma, brain cells are damaged and die. This damage does not normally show any visible signs of slowing down or memory loss at first. This happens slowly through the years, until it is almost too late. This lack of concentration or memory loss makes it hard to perform mental tasks.

Neuroplasticity happens through proper nutrition, physical exercise and brain exercises. As your brain cells and neurotransmitters are created and strengthened, you start to build up your 'cognitive reserves' or the brains ability to withstand damage due to aging, stress and other factors.

Researchers now believe that if you will implement a brain-healthy lifestyle and exercise your brain you can increase your brain's cognitive reserves. This is just like adding weight training for your muscles and building them up to help you retain more muscles as you get older.

Here is a short list from a very long list of idea to give your brain a workout that goes beyond a healthy diet and normal physical exercise:

- Learn Music – Join a choir or learn to play a musical instrument.
- Learn A Language – This can be sign language or a foreign language. Make sure it is something you can use with people who live around you. It will make learning easier and fun.
- Start a new hobby that involves fine-motor skills which help refine your hand-eye capabilities. This could include drawing, painting, assembling a puzzle or knitting. You get the idea.
- Use your other hand. Brush your teeth or any other task with the 'other hand' or non-dominant hand.
- Break out of your Routine. Switch up your morning activities or other parts of your daily routine. Drive to or from work a different way.

Your brain is like your body – it does not function well in a boring, non-stimulating routine. So for your brains sake – mix it up a bit.

Bonus Tip!

Rewire your brain for Happiness – Take In and Enjoy the Good in Life

I know that you encounter a few positive moments throughout each day. Many of these moments are small or seem to be insignificant, but they can be critical in changing your perspective and how the brain works. To do this you must take the time to;

- Appreciate the positive moments – moments of joy, happiness
- Increase the Intensity and Duration of these moments in your mind

We do this by lingering on them longer. Enjoy the moment and really feel the joy and happiness of experience. This is very effective in helping the brain to 'rewire' itself from a natural bias toward negativity to a more positive bias.

Researchers tell us now that when you appreciate and maximize the small, positive experiences, "...increasingly there's a sense of being filled up already inside, or already feeling safe inside, or already feeling loved and liked and respected. So we have less of a sense of striving... Insecurity falls away because you've got the good stuff inside of yourself.

"The more that things seem fresh and new, the more that you're looking at them with a beginner's mind or child's mind, that's going to increase brain structure because the brain is always looking for what's new."

So, break the routine and do things a little different every day AND linger longer on the positive experiences that you have throughout your day and you will have a strong, healthy and happy brain.

ACTION ITEM: Change up your daily routine –
drive to work a different way, brush your teeth with
the 'other' hand. Mix things up a little.

Take an extra minute or to think about and
appreciate, all the little positive experiences, thoughts
or moments. This will help the brain grow more
'positive' neurons.

27. DAILY WALKS - BungyPump Walking

Going on daily walks has been promoted by health care professionals for years. You may have taken an occasional walk through your neighborhood. There are indeed health benefits from leisure walks. But if you want to spice up those walks a little bit you have to try BungyPump walking.

These special walking poles were developed a few years ago and are manufactured in Sweden. These poles have quickly spread across Europe and they are now in the U.S.

BungyPump fitness poles help transform a normal walk or easy hike into a complete body workout that will exercise 90% of your muscles. Compared to going on a normal walk, these fitness poles will burn up to 77% more calories. You know that burning calories leads to weight loss.

They have rigid or solid walking sticks used in Nordic Walking or hiking. The BungyPump poles have a featured 'built-in suspension system', that provides smooth and steady resistance every time the poles are pressed down, without any straining or jarring movements.

The pole height is adjustable. The poles come with different amounts of resistance. They vary from 8, 13, and 22 pounds.

The 8 pound resistance is for beginners. The 22 pounder is for seasoned athletes or very active individuals.

Watch these informative videos to see the BungyPump™ in action. (http://thehealthybabyboomer.com/bungypump/)

Mile for mile, using the BungyPump is 30% more efficient than walking without them. It is fun and enjoyable. I love mine. Put the 'spring' back into your walks and watch your body tone up and moods soar.

ACTION ITEM: Check the link above and find out more about the BungyPumps and see them in action. Then go out for a walk.

28. STRENGTH TRAINING

Strength Training: *A type of physical exercise specializing in the use of resistance to induce muscular contraction which builds strength, anaerobic endurance, and size of skeletal muscles.*

When it comes to your muscles - USE IT OR LOSE IT!

Not all types of exercises are designed to build and strengthen muscles. Some like aerobics are designed to burn calories and build your cardiovascular system. You need to build up your muscles and keep them toned for your older years.

Here is a short list of benefits of strength training:

- Helps control your weight. Muscles are more efficient at burning calories than any other part of your body. So the more toned your muscles, the easier it is to control your weight.
- Provides similar improvements in depression as anti-depressant medications. When you participate in strength training programs, your self-confidence and self-esteem improve, which has a strong impact on your overall quality of life and happiness.

- Helps develop strong bones. By stressing your bones, strength training increases bone density and reduces the risk of osteoporosis.
- Sharpen your focus and mind. Some research suggests that regular strength training helps improve attention and memory for older adults.
- Helps boost your stamina. As you get stronger, you won't fatigue as easily. Building muscle also contributes to better balance.
- Manage chronic conditions. This can help reduce the symptoms of many chronic conditions, including back pain, arthritis, obesity, heart disease and diabetes.

Strength Training can be done at a gym or you can easily do them in the privacy of your own home. There are 4 common types of strength training:

1. Body Weight - Basically you are using your body as the weights or resistance. These would be exercises like squats, crunches, planks, pushups, etc. There are hundreds of variations of these types of strength training.
2. Resistance Tubing – Resistance tubing is inexpensive, light weight and come in many different types and resistance levels. Found in most sporting goods stores.
3. Free Weights or Weight Lifting – This is the most commonly thought of strength training. This type uses barbells and dumbbells.
4. Weight Machines – Most gyms and fitness centers offer different resistance or weight lifting machines. You can even buy them for home use.

So add some strength or resistance training into your exercise schedule for a happier and healthier life.

ACTION ITEM: Experiment with some of the different types of strength or resistance training to see which one you like. Then start doing strength training 2-3 times a week.

29. BOUNCE FOR YOUR HEALTH - Cellerciser

REBOUNDING – The Total Body Workout!

You may not be familiar with Rebounding or the Cellerciser™. A Rebounder is a mini-trampoline. A Cellerciser™ is a top of the line Rebounder that is made of the highest quality materials and special patented springs.

The Cellerciser™ has been helping change the way individuals exercise for over 20 years. Tens of thousands of people have had their health improved during this time. People of all ages love to use the Cellerciser™, including myself and my grandchildren.

Regular exercise (bouncing) on a Cellerciser™ or rebounder helps to strengthen all of your 75 trillion cells beyond their current capacity. Using this rebounder flexes each cell up to 100 times per minute and improves every joint, muscle and body system. When your cells are very healthy, all the body systems operate better and the entire body benefits.

Rebounding utilizes all 5 types of exercises at once for a complete and total workout.

ISOTONIC   AEROBIC
ISOMETRIC

According to different research, using a Cellerciser™ can burn calories:

11 times faster than Walking

5 times faster than Swimming

3 times faster than Running

These results were achieved in as little as 10 minutes of bouncing a day! There is a long list of benefits that have been documented after a ton of research.

Rebound your way to a happy and healthy life.

ACTION ITEM: Research Rebounding and especially the Cellerciser™ and see if it is right for you.

SPIRITUALITY:

30. WHAT DOES SPIRITUALITY MEAN TO YOU? DEFINE IT!

"Those who have a strong spiritual foundation tend to heal quicker and are generally healthier, both in mind and body, compared to those who do not have spirituality in their lives."

This statement comes from personal experience and training, many scientific studies, and the experience of thousands of health practitioners and health coaches. The research is there to support this opening statement, if one will put forth the time to look for it. But first you need to define what spirituality means to you.

'Spirituality can be a broad concept that has room for different perspectives. Generally speaking, it includes a sense of connection or close association with something much bigger than you, and it generally involves a search for meaning in life. It is something that touches all of us and as such is a universal human experience.'

Spirituality has different meanings to different people. But before you can improve or strengthen your spirituality you must be able to define it – for you. I know what it means to me, and for me it includes being active in my religious community or church.

Here is a couple of different concepts or ideas of spirituality.

1. Non-religious or secular individuals see spirituality as nothing more than, 'an inner path enabling a person to

discover the essence of his/her being...aspects of life and human experience which go beyond a purely materialistic view of the world without necessarily accepting belief in a supernatural reality or divine being.'

2. Christians and other religions reject the previous idea of spirituality. I fall into this group. Spirituality among Christians and others vary widely, but have one thing in common – it involves our relationship, to some level, with a personal creator, or God who exists outside of us and has revealed himself to us at some level.

3. Spirituality - includes the body, mind, soul and relationships or in other words, the whole person. It also includes all aspects of your life, and is a lived experience. Think of it as a journey throughout your life that involves the elements of values and beliefs. These elements help motivate you to grow, develop and expand your life; causing a transformation of your consciousness and thus your life. This can involve the knowing and experiencing God, not just knowing about God or the higher power of the Universe.

You might find yourself in one of these areas or a combination. Either way, your health and happiness can really be affected by your level of spirituality. Your body, mind and spirit will love you if you will strengthen your spirituality.

ACTION ITEM: Ponder about Spirituality in your life and define it for you, then do something to strengthen spirituality in your daily life.

31. WHAT IS MY LIFE PURPOSE?

You must develop a strong sense of who you are and what your purpose is here on this earth. Depression, anxiety, or having poor health can suck the life out of you; leaving you feeling like your life is pointless. In general, life can seem empty and meaningless at times, even if you are in pretty good shape. Questions about the meaning of life are a profound issue that is facing all of humanity.

There is no one right answer or predetermined meaning to life that applies to you and everyone else. It is up to you to find the answers and it is also up to you to make your life meaningful and have a purpose. Nobody can do it for you! When it comes to societies and communities, everyone will have to find how best to work together to build meaningful futures.

It is very important that you have a strong core belief system and to really understand this belief system as to how it relates to your purpose of life. If you do, then when those dark days come into your life, you will know who you are and what your purpose or mission is.

Emily Deans, M.D., a well-seasoned and experienced clinician had this to say,

"Religion and Spirituality are an important part of many people's lives, and in my experience, it can lend significant benefits in resiliency (resistant to future episodes). I've seen non-spiritual folk struggle more, perhaps, with feelings they are unloved and unworthy when traumatized than those with a spiritual "back-up" who feel that, no matter what happens, they have a spiritual connection to something greater. In addition, the spiritual and religious don't seem to wrestle as much with those existential questions of 'why am I here? What is my purpose?' that can plague the non-spiritual."

For your own peace of mind, you need to decide, <u>for yourself</u>, what you are supposed to accomplish while you are alive on this planet. When you can answer this question, you will be more at peace within yourself and with all those people around you, and your life will have much more meaning and purpose.

ACTION ITEM: On deep spiritual topics you need to take time to do some deep soul searching. Take some time to ponder this question – What is my purpose in life? What is my mission (what am I to accomplish) in this life?

32.   WHERE DID I COME FROM? - IS THERE LIFE AFTER DEATH?

These questions have been pondered, debated and the answers even fought over since the beginning of time. But if you can study, ponder and come to an understanding of what these answers mean to you, life will have greater meaning.

Wikipedia had this to say – Pre-existence, Beforelife, Pre-mortal Existence refers to the belief that each individual human soul or spirit existed before mortal conception, and at some point before birth, this spirit or soul enters or is placed into the body. Concepts of pre-existence can encompass either the belief that the soul came into existence at some time prior to conception or the belief that the soul is eternal.

Only you can decide what you believe deep down in your heart and soul. I just encourage you to think about it and ponder these deep but very meaningful and impactful questions. Did your soul live before you were born? Do you believe in a life after death or do you believe that once you take your last breath it is all over?

I feel the way you answer these two questions is very important to your long term mental wellbeing, and how you approach the trials that you face in this life. It is very comforting to me, to know that my spirit existed before being born on this earth, that there is a God and that I have a purpose here in this life and especially that there is life after this mortal life.

When you discover the answers for yourself, life will take on a new meaning and you will then be able to find true peace and happiness in your life.

ACTION ITEM: Ponder, meditate or pray and if you can answer the questions – Where did I come from? Is there life after death?

33. PRACTICE THANKFULNESS

Think it, Feel it, Do it.

Did you know people are not hardwired to be grateful? So to develop Thankfulness and have it part of your life, it is going to require practice, daily practice.

Thankfulness comes in three stages:

      1st   Recognition – Initial thought

2nd   Acknowledgement – Yes indeed, <u>it</u> is good

3rd   Appreciation – Better than the alternatives

Gratitude or Thankfulness is a thought process. It might only take a second or two to run through the three stages.

According to research and studies, practicing Thankfulness has some very positive side effects, such as:

- Strengthens Relationships and makes you a better friend. According to a 2003 study, gratitude or thankfulness can boost pro-social behaviors, such as helping other people who have problems or lending emotional support to another person.
- Strengthens Mental Health, especially in teenagers. People are happier, have a more positive outlook on life, and have more hope than those who do not practice Thankfulness.
- Better Sleep for those who took 15 minutes prior to going to bed and wrote down things they were thankful for.
- Improves Health including strengthening the immune system, and the heart. Studies showed that feelings of appreciation and positive emotions slowed the heart rate and fewer cases of sickness.

There are a number of ways to implement and increase more Gratitude or Thankfulness into your daily life. Here are three ideas you can work on today.

1. Give at least one compliment every day. This can be a compliment to a person or you can ask someone to share your appreciation of something. (I appreciate _____, don't you?)
2. Make a promise with yourself not to criticize, gossip or complain for 7-10 day. If you slip up, that is OK, just start

over. Take notice of all the energy you spend if a negative thought comes up.

3. Offer a Prayer of Thanks. In a 2007 poll 70% of those surveyed (all religions combined) said they pray daily. Studies show that those who say 'Thank You' more often than "please give me..." experience a higher level of satisfaction in life!

So now that you know about Thankfulness and how beneficial it is to your relationships, health (both physical and mental) and overall wellness, it is time to implement it into your daily life. When you are more thankful for the big and little things in life the healthier and happier you will be.

ACTION ITEM: Everyday, share with another person, at least one compliment about something you are thankful for.

34. PRAYER

"Prayer is the key of the morning and the bolt of the evening."
— Mahatma Gandhi

A PRAYER is a 'solemn request for help or an expression of thanks that is addressed to God or an object of worship.' It is also an 'earnest hope or wish'.

Man has been praying since Adam and Eve and as long as man has been able to ponder his existence and life. There is no established evidence that God or a Higher Power actually 'hears' your prayers but in recent years there is mounting evidence that prayer has measurable effects on your life and health.

Based on personal experience, I know that God hears and answers my prayers. Let's find out what the results are of some of the many research studies done on prayer and health. Prayer helps:

- Helps reduce stress – both physical and mental. Prayer evens out your emotional reaction to stress.
- Reduces your chance of suffering from anxiety and depression.
- Makes you nicer and reduces feelings of aggression.
- You become more forgiving.
- Increases your levels of dopamine, thus increasing your happiness level.
- Increase humility, less greedy for money and material things and just a better person.
- You live longer.

The results will depend on your expectations of receiving results. According to researchers from Baylor University, people who pray to a loving and protective God are less likely to experience anxiety-related disorders such as worry, fear, self-consciousness, social anxiety and obsessive compulsive behavior, compared to people who pray but don't really expect to receive any comfort or protection from God. So expect results and you will get results.

Prayer can be a mighty tool for healing, comfort and to boost your mood. Add daily prayer into your life and you will see wonderful changes in your health and happiness.

ACTION ITEM: If you do not pray, start by praying once a day for a week and see if you don't see and feel a difference in your life. If you do pray, try working on your 'expectations' and see if things improve.

35. MEDITATION

For thousands of years people in different cultures have used some form of meditation. Originally it was used to help people improve their understanding of sacred and mystical forces in life. In the modern Western cultures meditation is more commonly used to reduce stress by achieving a more relaxed state. But meditation is equally powerful in developing or increasing ones spirituality.

Since meditation is used primarily as a spiritual tool in the different countries of origin, it has been put within the category of spirituality. The nice thing about meditation is that once implemented into your daily routine it will accomplish two major goals at once – stress management and spiritual growth.

Researchers at Harvard Medical School found that, in long-term meditation practitioners, far more 'disease-fighting genes' were switched on and active, compared to those who did not practice meditation.

Dr. Herbert Benson, lead researcher, said, 'We found a range of disease-fighting genes were active in the relaxation practitioners that were not active in the control group.' Then the researchers ask the control group to start a daily meditation practice. 'After two months, their bodies began to change; the genes that help fight inflammation, kill diseased cells and protect the body from cancer all began to switch on.'

They also found that with regular meditation the positive healthy effect kept increasing. In other words the more people practiced meditation the greater their chances were of remaining free of disease and developed a stronger immune system.

Other laboratory studies have found that meditation produced positive changes in the brain circuits involving the regulation of emotions and the reduction of the stress hormone cortisol.

Meditation clears the 'monkey mind' and helps you be in the present moment and focus on just one thing. Meditation along with prayer can greatly influence and improve your spirituality while reducing your stress levels. Improve in both those areas and you will find more peace, harmony, health and happiness in your life. Meditate today!

ACTION ITEM: Try different types of meditation and find one you enjoy and do it daily for a week.

36. CREATE A GRATITUDE JOURNAL

Your gratitude journal does not have to be fancy or formal; it can be a simple notebook. It is up to you. What really matters is that you write in it on a regular basis – keep it where you can review it, especially on those down days.

So what do you put in a gratitude journal? Everything you are thankful for! Write down one or two things or experiences that you are grateful for without duplications. You can list a couple of things that happened during the day that impressed you or what you learned from an experience.

Here are just a few reasons to start writing in a Gratitude Journal.

- o Improves your sleep – According to researchers if you spend 15 minutes before bedtime, writing and pondering things you are grateful for, you should fall asleep quicker, stay asleep longer and sleep deeper.
- o Improves attitude and may turn you into an optimist – Attitudes improve and you become more optimistic after writing in a gratitude journal and pondering over the list. Optimistic attitudes increase your overall physical, mental and emotional health.
- o The body feels every thought – Thinking about positive things and writing down things and experiences that you are thankful for helps the body and mind relive those positive moments.
- o Letting Go of limiting beliefs – You are your own worst critic. You tend to see what you expect in life and those expectations are limited by your beliefs. If you can start to change those beliefs about yourself, your life will start to change.

Your future will thank you for it – In 10 to 20 years from now you will be a different person, if you keep up a gratitude journal during that whole time. I think that you will feel healthier, happier, less stressed, more vibrant and just more fun to be around. Try to prove me wrong – keep writing in the gratitude journal for 10 years then look back and see if you are not a different and better person than when you started. I dare you!

ACTION ITEM: Start your Gratitude Journal. Write in it every night or at least once a week. Just list 1 or 2 things you are thankful for.

STRESS MANAGEMENT:

37. SLEEP - A Time For Renewal

Did you know that during deep sleep your body renews itself by repairing muscles and tissues as well as build up your energy supplies for the next day? This is also the time when your body undergoes a detox – the body rids itself of toxins from all the different systems.

Adults need between 7 ½ and 9 hours of sleep **every** night in order to maintain good health. This may be impossible for some people. But know that consistency is the key-and cutting back on sleep can have more harmful effects than you know.

According to medical literature it is becoming more and more evident that every tissue, cell and body system benefits from adequate sleep and rest. So the most effective thing you can do to restore and maintain a healthy brain, body and mind is to get 8-9 hours of sleep.

There are huge volumes of studies that show that if you consistently get less sleep you are more likely to develop health problems that range from high blood pressure, obesity, depression, anxiety and other negative consequences.

Do you suffer from brain fog or memory lapses? During sleep your brain goes through a process called 'memory consolidation'. This is when the new information that was learned during the day is put into the memory banks. The brain also replenishes neurotransmitters which includes dopamine and serotonin – which elevates your mood during the day.

It is vitally important for proper brain health, memory and mood, that you get enough sleep. Getting enough sleep is another great way to take care of your body, mind and spirit, so please get enough sleep.

ACTION ITEM: Calculate backwards and figure out what time you have to be in bed each night in order to get 8 hours of sleep. Write it down and work hard to be in bed on time, no matter what. Your health depends on it.

38. DEEP BREATHING EXERCISE

Breathing correctly is not only important for living longer but also in being in a good mood and to keep performing at your best.

Deep breathing is a simple but powerful relaxation technique that focuses on full, deep and relaxed breaths. These deep breaths deliver the following benefits:

- ❖ A quick way to reduce your stress levels
- ❖ Breathing Elevates Moods
- ❖ Breathing Boosts Energy levels and Improves Stamina
- ❖ Breathing Detoxifies and Releases Toxins
- ❖ Breathing Relieves Pain
- ❖ Breathing Strengthens the Immune System
- ❖ It is very easy to learn
- ❖ It can be done almost anywhere
- ❖ The cornerstone of many other relaxation practices

❖ Can be combined with other relaxation elements such as music and aromatherapy
❖ It just takes a few minutes and a relaxing, quiet place.

Here is a simple deep breathing technique to help you get started. There are many different techniques available. Most all deep breathing techniques use your abdomen instead of your chest.

EQUAL BREATHING

Step #1 -   INHALE through the nose for a count of four (4). Your stomach should rise. Balance within the body is a good thing and it all starts with the breath.

Step #2 -   EXHALE through the nose for a count of four (4). Your stomach should contract. This adds a slight, natural resistance to the breath.

Step #3 -   Repeat steps #1 and #2 for 2-5 minutes or until you are relaxed.

Breathing deeply from the abdomen is the key. This allows you to get more fresh air into your lungs. You inhale more oxygen when you take deep breaths using the abdomen instead of using your upper chest. You will feel less anxious and less tension when you are getting more oxygen into your system.

Deep Breathing can be done anywhere and anytime. The benefits are great and your moods will improve and your health and energy levels will improve. Try it!

ACTION ITEM: Learn simple deep breathing techniques so when you need to de-stress or need a quick energy boost you can just start breathing!

39.   *Yesterday - TODAY - Tomorrow*

**"Yesterday is in the Past, Tomorrow may never
come, Today is Now.
Live Life Today."**

Too many people live in the past. If you are always worried about what you did or did not do in the past you can easily slip into anxiety or depression. You need to realize that yesterday is in the past and you can't live in the past all the time and stay emotionally and physically healthy. You can't change yesterday so learn from yesterday and make changes Today so you don't repeat the yesterdays.

Tomorrow never comes. Do you live in tomorrow? Do you wish your life away – 'I can't wait until Saturday'. Many people spend so much time worrying about tomorrow or another day in the future, that they miss out on Today. Again, if you spend much of your time thinking and worrying about tomorrow you will become discouraged, maybe depressed or suffer from anxiety. You need to forget about tomorrow.

Today is Now. Make the best of today because it will soon be gone and you can never get it back. When these 24 hours are gone they are gone. This very moment should be the most important moment in your life. You need to make the most of it. Those people who seem to be able to live in the moment or today, seem to be less stressed, happier, healthier and more at peace.

ACTION ITEM: If there is something in the past that you worry about, then resolve it and move on. Enjoy the moment today. Smell the smells around you. Embrace the warmth of the sun. Do what you need to do to BE in the moment and in Today. Tomorrow will take care of itself.

40.   GUIDED VISUALIZATION

"What the mind of man can <u>conceive</u> and <u>believe,</u> it can <u>achieve</u>"

Napoleon Hill

A guided visualization usually consists of soft, beautiful and relaxing music and a male or female guide. This guide will first gently talk you through a deep breathing exercise to get you relaxed. Second, the guide will verbally take you to a wonderful, peaceful place. It could be a beach, in a forest or some place in the universe. Once there, the guide will give you positive statements or re-enforcements on whatever subject you are working on. Then the guide will take you back to where you started your visualization journey. When you are finished you should be feeling relaxed and at peace.

The real power of guided visualizations or meditations is in the use of your imagination and visualization to train the brain and subconscious mind. Your subconscious mind then creates positive changes in your personal life. This is one of the main advantages of guided visualization and why guided mediations can be more powerful than passive, traditional meditations.

This type of meditation helps you to experience positive, vivid images in your mind that either directly or symbolically represent whatever changes you want to make in your life.

You are in such a deep state of relaxation, during a guided meditation, that the images your guide describes can become very vivid and alive. When you immerse yourself in a guided visualization session and you listen to the positive suggestions, it becomes a peaceful and powerful experience and the results are real and almost immediate. You will feel so much better, physically, emotionally, mentally and also spiritually.

ACTION ITEM: Obtain a high quality Guided Visualization CD and use it every day for a week and see how you feel.

41. KIRTAN KRIYA (Saa-Taa-Naa-Maa)

Kirtan Kriya – (KEER-tun, KREE-a) is a meditation from the Kundalini yoga tradition and has been practiced for thousands of years. This meditation is sometimes called a singing exercise because it involves singing the sounds – Saa, Taa, Naa, Maa as you do a repetitive finger movement.

This is a non-religious practice and can be adapted to several lengths of time, but studies have shown that doing it for just 12 minutes a day, reduce stress levels and increases brain activity in the area that controls memory. Those who have memory problems, such as Alzheimer's disease, have found help performing this mediation daily.

How to practice Kirtan Kriya

1. While sitting with your spine straight and your eyes closed, and cross-legged (if you are flexible enough) repeat singing the Saa, Taa, Naa, Maa sounds. As you sing each sound, visualize the sound flowing in through the top of your head and out the middle of your forehead.
2. For the first two minutes, sing the sounds in your normal voice.
3. For the second two minutes, sing the sounds in a whisper.
4. For the next 4 minutes, sing the sounds silently to yourself.
5. Then reverse the order and whisper the sounds for two minutes and then out loud for two minutes.
The total time: 12 minutes
6. To come out of or to finish the meditation, inhale very deeply, stretch your hands high above your head, and then bring them down slowly in a sweeping motion as you exhale.

The Finger movements (on both hands) while singing the sounds per the instructions above.

Saa – Touch thumbs to index fingers
Taa – Touch thumbs to middle fingers
Naa – Touch thumbs to ring fingers
Maa – Touch thumbs to little fingers

This is a very simple meditation, after you have practiced it a couple of times. This is a great mental health exercise. Your body, mind and spirit will reward you for implementing Kirtan Kriya into your weekly schedule.

ACTION ITEM: Do a web search for Kirtan Kriya and find a video showing you how to do this meditation. Try Kirtan Kriya a couple of times a week and see if you can feel a difference after each session. If so, add it into you weekly routines.

42. MONTHLY MASSAGE

Most people think of pampering and relaxation when they think of massages. This part is true but research is finding that massages are as good as many medications for many health issues. Plus there are plenty of preventative health properties to regular massages.

Massage can be a great tool to have in your 'stay healthy toolbox'. It can be a tool to help take charge of your well-being and overall health. You can even learn how to do self-massage or how to do massages at home with a spouse. You can do a massage for many different reasons including some of the following:

Eases muscle pains – according to the Annals of Internal Medicine a massage is as effective as other methods of relieving chronic back pain.

Soothes depression and anxiety – according to the International Journal of Neuroscience, women who were diagnosed with breast cancer, who received a massage three times a week were less angry and depressed than those who did not have the massages.

Improves Sleep – you know how important it is to your health to get enough good, quality sleep. Massages help your body and mind relax so that you can fall asleep easier.

Strengthens the Immune system – according to the Journal of Alternative and Complementary Medicine, a massage increases your white blood cells which plays a major role in protecting the body against diseases.

Relieves Headaches – The Granada University (in Spain) did a study and found that a single massage session has immediate effect on pain levels from chronic tension headaches.

Whatever the reason, your health may improve greatly with a monthly massage. So schedule a monthly massage with your local massage therapist. Your body, mind and spirit will really appreciate the boost.

ACTION ITEM: Schedule time each month for a massage!! Pamper yourself for a change.

43.   MUSIC - Calming and Healing

Music has always been an important part of every culture and society because of its healing powers and influence on the body, mind and spirit. There are some modern music that is detrimental to the mind, body and spirit. You know the music when you hear it. You start to feel your body tense up, heart rate increases and your head starts to pound. Choose your music wisely.

There are a lot of studies that show certain music has therapeutic traits. Let's take a look at some of them:

Pain Relief – Many studies have shown that if you listen to Classical music such as Mozart, Beethoven or Bach you can have relief from your muscle pain. Other calm, slow music has also been shown to help with pain. It only takes about 25 minutes a day for

10-14 days to help relieve back pain and as a side benefit – helps you sleep better.

Improved Memory – Research now shows that people who have memory loss respond best by listening to music of their choice (music from their childhood or early adult years). New research shows that memory was improved with those Alzheimer's patients who listened to music that they were very familiar with. Music can bring back memories from the past.

Control Your Heart Rate and Breathing – You can control your body, to a degree, simply by choosing the music that you listen to. A slow, meditative tempo has a relaxing effect on your body by slowing down your heart rate and breathing. Listening to faster music with an upbeat tempo speeds up your breathing and heart rate. So again pick your music wisely.

Increase Learning and Memorization – There have been hundreds of studies that have proven that just by listening to classical music like Bach, Beethoven and Mozart learning increases substantially. Memorization becomes much easier when done listening to a Mozart Concerto. So when you need to learn something quickly, play classical music when you study. You will be amazed.

Your problems become easier – Music helps you to express your emotions. It is called 'Melodic Encouragement' that helps you to let go of suppressed feelings and emotions. Music can help you release those suppressed feelings. If you cry, that's OK. Tears represent feelings that must be expressed. As they say, 'Feeling is Healing.'

Soft, relaxing music has medicinal properties and can elevate moods. Use music to relax and heal.

ACTION ITEM: This week listen to different soft classical or new age music and find several you like. Listen to them several times a week. Music soothes the savage beast within.

44.   WRITE IT DOWN

We are talking about using a pen or pencil and a piece of paper. According to research the actual writing down of information helps you to better retain that information. It is the physical act of writing that sends signals from your hand to your brain that builds motor memory. These motor memories are more easily retained and for longer periods of time.

Not only is writing beneficial for memory retention, it has many other health benefits such as:

Speed Healing By Expressing Written Emotions – In a New Zealand study it was discovered that those individuals who wrote in a journal about their deepest, most innermost thoughts and feelings had quicker healing of skin biopsies.

Helps Improve Attitude During Stressful Times – In a 2008 study, Cancer patients were asked to do "Expressive Writing" (express their fears, hopes and dreams). The results found that this helped the cancer patients think about their disease in a different way, but it also improved their quality of life.

Improve Self-Love – Write a Love Letter To Yourself – As weird as this sounds, writing a love letter to yourself is a great way to feel better about yourself. Write a letter explaining all the good qualities you see in yourself. It is OK to pat yourself on the back once in a while. You have to love yourself before you can truly love someone else.

Goals Are Easier To Achieve –The old adage; 'A goal not written is only a wish' is very true. Write down your goals – be specific and give them a time frame. Some goals can just be put on a 'bucket list' and forgotten – but somehow they still come to pass. There is just something about writing goals down. Do it!

Forgiveness Letters – You can write a letter forgiving yourself or someone else that has offended or hurt you. Just doing the act of writing it all down helps the forgiving process.

Writing down happy memories, things you are grateful for, your fears or goals will help you retain the memories, overcome fears and help your life be healthier and happier.

ACTION ITEM: This week spend more time writing down your thoughts and feelings, both happy and sad, both loving and forgiving. Don't forget about your goals and dreams.

45. LAUGHTER

Laughter can bring people together and improve relationships and over-all health as well as anything else out there. It also creates one of the best feelings during and after laughter.

Doctors and researchers have found that people who have a positive outlook on life and laughter helps fight disease better than people who do not laugh much and tend to be more negative.

Laughter can increase your overall sense of well-being by having the following benefits:

Boost Immune System – Your T cells are immediately activated and begin to help you fight off sickness and disease. T cells are very specialized immune system cells that are just waiting in your body for activation. When you start to feel sick start to laugh and watch the cold or flu start to diminish.

Chronic Pain – Laughing helps your body to release endorphins, which can help ease chronic pain. Aching joints start to feel better during and after laughter.

Improves Mood – Laugh out loud if you want to lighten the mental load. Cortisol (stress hormone) levels are lowered in the body and also the levels of endorphins are increased, which help boost your mood. Research studies support laughter as a great way to break the downward spiral to depression.

Tones Up The Abs – Laughter can help you tone your abs. When you are laughing, the muscles in your stomach expand and contract, which is similar to when you intentionally exercise your abs. So add laughter to your daily exercise routine for firmer abs.

Laughter has shown benefits within the physiological, psychological, social, spiritual, and quality-of-life areas of life. Therapeutic effectiveness of laughter can be derived from either spontaneous laughter (triggered by external stimuli or positive emotions) or self-induced laughter (triggered by oneself at will). Your brain is not able to distinguish between these two types. Benefits may be achieved with one or the other. Laughter is Laughter, so just laugh!

ACTION ITEM: This week watch a funny movie, sitcom or read jokes, anything that will make you laugh out loud. See how you feel after.

PART 2 - SECONDARY FOODS

46. REPLACE THE BAD WITH GOOD - REPLACE THE GOOD WITH BETTER

This is a very easy 'first step' in changing from the SAD – Standard American Diet – to a healthier diet. You do not have to make major radical diet changes overnight. It can be done on a slower, more gradual change. It is all about the journey, not perfection.

So the idea here is to take one unhealthy food from your diet and replace it with something better. You can do this once a week. Then you can replace the good items with something better.

Example: Regular hamburger (bad – high fat content) to Lean Hamburger (good – lower fat content). Then you can change from the good hamburger to Grass Fed Beef Hamburger (Better – low fat, no antibiotics and hormones, not gmo corn fed).

Fruit juices (bad) - whole fruit (good) – organic fruit (better/best).   You get the idea!

You are what you eat so upgrade the quality of your food when you can. Start with getting rid of the highly processed foods and go to whole foods then move on to organic where you can.

ACTION ITEM: Each week remove 1 unhealthy, highly processed food from your diet and replace it with a whole food, healthier version, and where possible go with organic. When it comes to meat go with grass fed.

47. THE 90/10 DIET RULE

Changing diets for health reasons or for weight loss can be a daunting task. Many people think that when they 'go on a diet' to lose weight that they must be perfect. They consider it a 'deprivation' diet. Weight loss is a journey not perfection. Changing from the Standard American Diet to a healthier diet does take some work.

Keep one thing in mind. It is OK to have a 'treat' once in a while. Sometimes we slip up and eat that piece of cake, or have some of that 'white pasta' or slice of pizza. It is not the end of the weight loss journey.

Here is a good rule to base your diet on:

Eat Healthy 90% Of The Time –Treat Yourself 10%

This means that if you slip up once in a while it is not the end of the world. Here is the best part of this rule. IF you do really well on eating right all week then you can have that little splurge (couple of cookies, slice of pie, or whatever) on the weekend.

In other words, it is OK to slip up or have a little treat once a week, without wrecking your entire diet or feeling guilty. It will get easier with time. Experiment with different healthy dessert recipes until you find a couple that you like.

P.S. You don't need to be too fanatical with the healthy eating thing. This can be a turn off to family and friends. It is more important to stick to eating healthy, whole foods 90+% of the time than to stress out over eating perfect 100% of the time.

ACTION ITEM: This week try to eat healthy 90% of the time (whole foods) and when you do, give yourself a little reward. It is not about perfection, it's about the journey.

48. THE CROWDING OUT METHOD

One of the best solutions to overcome cravings and giving up your favorite unhealthy foods is by using the – Crowding Out Method.

The Crowding Out Method – Eat and Drink the foods that are good for you early in the day and you will leave less room and minimize your desire for the unhealthy foods and drinks. Eating healthy foods can and will crowd out the junk food.

Vegetables are high in vitamins and minerals. You can eat a lot of them without gaining weight. As you increase the amount of vegetables, such as dark leafy greens, your body will not have as much room for the processed junk foods. Here is the nice thing about this; your body will naturally start to crave these healthy foods.

This works well when it comes to hydration. In the morning fill a water bottle with water and take it with you and sip it steadily throughout your morning. Refill it for the afternoon. Do this and it will leave less room for coffee, soda or alcohol and your body will respond better to the water.

The trick is to always have healthy foods and water available for snacks and when you are traveling. This will help you get through the day without impulsively eating junk food. This will take a little practice and planning, but it will be worth it. You will feel more energetic and happier. Crowding out the bad with the good works!!

ACTION ITEM: This week start increasing your intake of vegetables and water and see if you don't eat less processed junk food. Implement a 'Crowding Out'

49.   PURIFIED WATER - The Elixir Of Life

If you research history you will find that the civilizations that developed and maintained the purest and cleanest water supply were generally the strongest, most vibrant and healthiest societies of their time.

Many of the ancient civilizations used water as part of their medical treatments to heal injury and to treat many different diseases. These included the Greek, Persian, Hebrew, Chinese and Native American, to name a few.

Maintaining the proper level of body hydration is an essential part of your physiological functions. For example if the brain is not properly hydrated, your thinking ability becomes impaired, you start having problems making good decisions. You increase your chances of getting headaches and dizziness. If your liver becomes dehydrated it cannot break down fats and you can start to gain weight and your digestive system becomes imbalanced, and so on.

So it is vitally important that you keep your body properly hydrated. Since studies have shown that most people are under hydrated, you need to increase the amount of water that you drink each day.

Caution: Chlorine and Fluoride - There is a huge debate on whether chlorine and fluoride should be added into the water supply. The debate also includes discussion about if Chlorine and Fluoride cause cancer or not. I recommend removing them from your water by using a high quality water filter system.

Two Rules of Thumb: Drink 8 - 8 oz glasses of water a day.   Or ½ of your body weight in ounces. (weight = 150 lbs.   150 / 2 = 75 so drink 75 oz. of water)

Since each of you are different and unique, experiment with these two methods and see which works best for you. Your health will greatly improve just by making sure you get enough purified water into your body.   ***Drink more water!***

ACTION ITEM: Assess how much water you drink during an average day. Then increase that by 1-2 glasses and see how you feel.

50.   BE A COW NOT A CROC. - Chew Your Food

Have you watched a cow eat while grazing in a pasture? How do they eat? They are always chewing. They chew, chew, chew, chew and chew some more – then they swallow. They are slow eaters.

Have you been to the zoo when Crocodiles eat? So how do Croc's eat? You never see them chew their food. They chomp, chomp and swallow. They are fast eaters and practically swallow their food whole.

You should eat like a cow and not a croc! Some say chew 20 times and other say chew 50 times. You need to chew your food until it turns into liquid. Here are several reasons for chewing your foods more;

- Digestion actually starts with the chewing process. Digestion is improved with more chewing.
- Un-chewed foods can remain undigested and can cause bacteria overgrowth in the intestines.
- The chewing action and the production of saliva, sends a message to the stomach, intestines and to the whole gastrointestinal system that the digestion process has begun.
- The real flavors of plant foods are release only after they have been thoroughly chewed. This is also true with carbohydrates. The sweet flavors of these different foods become one of the rewards for eating and chewing.

Tip for chewing more –

- o Put your fork or spoon down between bites. This slows down the eating process and allows for more time to chew.

For better health and elevated moods – chew your foods like a cow and not a croc!

ACTION ITEM: For each meal that you eat today, slow down, chew your food completely and really enjoy the eating experience.

51. IS SUGAR TOXIC?

The short answer is YES! Many, many studies have found a connection between sugar consumption and many diseases and accelerated aging. Here are some facts and reasons for you to start today removing added sugars from your diet. Here are the facts:

Facts - 13% of the daily calories consumed by Americans come from added sugars in their foods. Based on this, you consume about 130 pounds of added sugar a year. That is equivalent to eating 22 teaspoons of added sugar a day! The American Heart Association said that the daily intake of added sugars for women must not exceed the equivalent of 6 teaspoons and for men they must not exceed 9.

Side Effects of exceeding these maximums;

- ✓ Causes the message that you are full, from your gut to your brain to misfire and causes your brain to think you are not full or that you have not eaten.
- ✓ The continual overeating of added sugar will speed up the browning effect of all your tissues caused by oxidative stress. In other words, your skin will age faster.
- ✓ Too much added sugar will irritate the lining of all your blood vessels which can impact the amount of oxygen that reaches all your different organs.
- ✓ When your liver receives an overdose of sugar, it has no choice but to turn the excess sugar into liver fat.
- ✓ Sugar triggers a Dopamine (a feel good neurotransmitter) response but when you eat too much sugar it starts to shut down the healthy signaling in the body. This means you have to eat more and more sugar in order to get that 'feel good feeling'.

Sugar is toxic to the body. All this added sugar to your food is slowly destroying your body. In order to live a long, healthy and happy life cut out most of the added sugars from your diet.

ACTION ITEM: Next time you go grocery shopping take time to read the food labels and only purchase foods with low sugar contents and without added sugars.

52. GLYCEMIC INDEX - Eat Low Glycemic Foods

"Not All Carbohydrate Foods Are Equal"

The Glycemic Index (GI) is a comparative ranking of carbohydrate in foods based on how they affect blood glucose levels. Some carbohydrates are digested and turned into sugar (blood glucose) at a slower rate than other carbs. So a food with a GI of 30 will turn to sugar at a much slower rate than a food with a GI of 95.

"The glycemic index (GI) is a ranking of carbohydrates on a scale from 0 to 100 according to the extent to which they raise blood sugar levels after eating. Foods with a high GI are those which are rapidly digested and absorbed and result in marked fluctuations in blood sugar levels. Low-GI foods, by virtue of their slow digestion and absorption, produce gradual rises in blood sugar and insulin levels, and have proven benefits for health. Low GI diets have been shown to improve both glucose and lipid levels in people with diabetes (type 1 and type 2). They have benefits for weight

control because they help control appetite and delay hunger. Low GI diets also reduce insulin levels and insulin resistance."
Glycemicindex.com

Here is a just a small sampling of foods with lower GI ratings and some with high GI ratings. Which foods are you eating?

LOWER GLYCEMIC FOODS	GI
Hummus (chickpea salad dip)	6
Grapefruit	25
Wheat Tortilla	30
Carrots (cooked)	35
Fettucini, average	32

HIGH GLYCEMIC FOODS	GI
Baked Russet Potato, average	111
Fruit Roll-ups	99
Bagel, White, Plain	95
Gatorade	78
Microwave popcorn, plain, average	55

ACTION ITEM: Look up some of the foods that you are currently eating and see how they rate on the Glycemic Food Index. Click here for a partial list. Change foods if you need to.

53. EAT MEAT 'SPARINGLY'

There is a lot of debate on how much meat we should be eating, from being Vegetarian / Vegan to the other end, eating the Paleo / Atkins diets. I feel we should be somewhere in the middle. We should follow the 'sparingly' guidelines followed by some religious groups.

Several religious groups have a scriptural basis for eating meat 'sparingly', if at all. Two of the more prominent groups are the Church of Jesus Christ of Latter-day Saints (The Word of Wisdom) and the Seventh Day Adventist. If you check their statistics they, as individual groups, have a much healthier and longer live span.

The definition of 'sparing' is left to each person's discretion. For me, I aim to get two-thirds of my protein from plants and just one-third from animal sources, or a 1:2 ratio. This is equivalent to three servings of meat (excluding two servings of fish/seafood) weekly.

A study done by Oxford University on the English diet, found that there was a reduction in the death rate from chronic diseases, when the meat intake was reduced to three servings a week. Three servings a week would be considered 'sparing'. These researchers projected that this change in diet would have the following benefits for England:

- 331,000 fewer deaths a year from heart diseases
- 9,000 fewer cancer deaths a year
- 5,000 fewer stroke deaths a year

Environmental Food Toxins and Pollution

According to another study, it is estimated that nearly 85% of your toxin exposure from foods, comes into your body from the meat you eat. These toxins come in the form of hormones, antibiotics, GMO's that are found in the food fed to the beef. You can reduce your expose by doing two things – reduce your consumption of meat and implement Secret #54.

So reduce your risk by reducing your consumption of beef and other meats in your diet and use meat as a flavoring in cooking. Implement this secret today for better health and happiness.

ACTION ITEM: Decide what 'sparingly' means to you and your family and try cutting your meat consumption down for a week or two and see how you feel.

54. MEAT - Grass Fed and Wild Caught

The Big Lie – *Meat is Meat is Meat* – It doesn't matter what the animal has been fed, the nutritional value is all the same. Here is the other part of the lie – The Hormones, anti-biotics and GMO foods given to the animals are not harmful to humans.

Research is proving the lie is correct. The difference between a grass-fed beef and a feed-lot fed beef is substantial. There is no comparison. Here are several advantages of grass-fed beef:
- o Contains 1/3 to 1/2 the amount of fat which means it will lower your LDL levels
- o Less Fats mean there are less calories
- o Contains 2-6 times that amount of Omega-3 fatty acids

○ Contains 4 times more vitamin E which helps reduce risk of cancer and heart disease

Free range Chickens produce eggs that contain as much as 20 times more Omega-3's than eggs from factory farms.

When it comes to fish and sea foods you want to only eat 'wild caught'. Much of the salmon sold in stores today come from fish farms. You have the same issues here as you do with the beef when it comes to anti-biotics and hormones. Now some farmed salmon are classified as GMO foods.

So when it comes to meat, go for quality. Go for 'Grass Feed', 'Wild Caught and Free Range' for your meat, fish and eggs. You will feel better and your moods may even soar.

ACTION ITEM: This week try eating some grass fed beef and cutting back on either the frequency or portion size of your meat and see how you feel.

55. BUY ORGANIC WHEN POSSIBLE

Go organic regardless of which diet you are on, even if you are on the SAD (Standard American Diet) plan. There is some debate on whether organic foods are worth the extra cost. You can make up your own mind. Here are several reasons why you will want to start adding in some organic foods into your diet.

♥ *More Nutrients* – Organics have more vitamins, minerals, micronutrients and enzymes than conventionally grown foods. Over 41 studies have shown the nutritional superiority of organically grown foods.

- ♥ *Reduce Chemical Toxins in the Body* – Did you know that there are currently over 600 different chemicals approved to use in commercially growing your foods? One study done by the National Academy of Science reported that 90% of these chemicals used have not been tested for long term health effects.

- ♥ *Avoid GMO foods* – To be labeled organic the food cannot be genetically modified. There is no mandatory GMO food labeling laws in the United States, so going with certified organic foods helps insure you are not eating GMO foods. Again there have been little long-term health studies done on GMO's.

- ♥ *Better Tasting* - Organically grown heirloom varieties of fruits and vegetables just plainly taste better. This is because the soil is well balanced and this helps grow strong, healthy plants.

These are just a few of the many different reasons eating organically grown fruits, vegetables and meats are a better choice over commercially grown foods. When you make the change to organic you will feel physically and mentally better. Try it!

ACTION ITEM: Try the Organic version of a few different foods and help your body and mind feel better.

56. THE CAFFEINE STRESS / DEPRESSION CONNECTION

Doctor Bruce McEwen said, *"Stress, or being stressed out, leads to behaviors and patterns that in turn can lead to a chronic stress burden and increase the risk of major depression."*

Studies are now showing that when you drink and eat caffeine it really does induce a state of stress within your body. Caffeine causes the adrenal glands to produce stress hormones that can and will remain in your blood stream up to 18 hours after you consume it.

Drinking a cup of coffee can give you a shot of caffeine strong enough to increase catecholamines or stress hormones. The stress turns on the cortisol (fight or flight hormone) switch along with insulin. Insulin causes and increases inflammation within the body and this in return causes you and your body to feel lousy.

Stress that is caused by caffeine can produce the following:

- Mood Swings (Depression / Anxiety)
- Insomnia
- Muscle Tension
- Impaired digestion
- Restrict Blood to the Brain
- Accelerate Heart Rate and Blood Pressure

Sometimes the stress response switch fails to shut off, because of chronic stress, and it can lead to depression and all the other issues listed above. It is imperative that this stress switch gets turned off.

The first thing you need to do is to cut back or eliminate caffeine from your diet – soda drinks, energy drinks, coffee and some teas. The second thing is to learn different techniques to help reduce and management all the other stress causing issues in your life.

ACTION ITEM: This week try to reduce the amount of caffeine in your diet and see if you feel less stressed.

57. WEEKLY DINNER MENU AND SHOPPING LIST

There are several benefits to having a weekly or monthly meal menu. Here are just a few:

1. It reduces a little stress and chaos in your life. Once the menu is set you know what you are going to fix.
    No looking at the cupboard and thinking, 'what am I going to fix.'
2. If you involve the family members in this meal planning process they will be less likely to complain when the meal is served.
3. You can have the recipes readily available beforehand.
4. Pre-prepared meal plans with menus take the guess work out of a weight-loss diet.

Here are a few benefits of having a menu-based shopping list:

1. Saves Time – You know what you need. You can get in and get out quickly.

2. Saves Money – Healthy foods are cheaper if you have a plan or list and stick to it.
3. It is a Plan – Saves you from wandering aimlessly down the aisles of the store wondering what to buy. You will buy junk food without a plan.
4. Stress Reducer – You know what you are going to fix for each meal and you have all the ingredients, therefore there are less last-minute glitzes at meal time.

If you can save time, money, reduce stress, eat more healthy meals and keep your sanity, all at the same time, why not develop a weekly or monthly meal plan and a shopping list to match. So for a stress free, healthy and happy life – plan your meals and shopping list ahead of time.

ACTION ITEM: This week sit down, with your family, and plan out all the meals for the week and put a shopping list together based on the meals and the recipes.

58. WHOLE GRAINS - Cereal

If you can tolerate grains (not gluten intolerant), the question then becomes how much grain should you be eating? According to a new study published in BMC Medicine, women who are eating about 1,800 calories should be eating about 53 grams of whole grains a day. For men it is slightly more.

When it comes to Cereal you must look for the word "Whole"_____. So when it comes to buying cereal the first ingredient should be 'whole-_____ flour.' Anything else means refined grains.

"When it comes to Whole Grain foods always follow this rule of thumb –

More Fiber than Sugar."

Here are some other helpful tips on finding healthy cereal.

1. FIBER – The more fiber the better. Do not settle for anything less than 3 grams per serving. The more fiber you can get in your cereal the longer you will feel full. Fiber is a must for healthy digestion and to keep you regular.
2. LIMIT SUGAR – Breakfast cereal is not a dessert! The low sugar in the cereal will help you avoid the sugar crash later on.
3. PROTEIN – Look for cereal with at least 5 grams of protein per serving. This will help you from overeating later. If your cereal meets all the other requirements but this one, just add an egg or yogurt to your meal.
4. READ THE INGREDIENT LIST – The first ingredient must be 'whole grain' and be limited to just a few ingredients, that you can pronounce and that sound like a food. Avoid highly processed foods.
5. PORTION SIZE – With cereal you may be tempted to eat more than one serving. Stick with the serving size for a few days and see how you feel. I think you will find that with the healthier whole grain cereals you will not need to eat as much.

Feel free to 'bulk' up your cereal with some chopped nuts or a little fruit. Adding more Whole Grains into your diet will help you feel healthier and happier – IF you can tolerate the grains. Try adding more grains to your diet and see if you start to feel happier and healthier.

ACTION ITEM: When you go shopping this week search out and try a healthier 'whole grain' cereal. Also look for other ways to increase whole grains into your diet.

59.   WHOLE GRAINS - Bread

Just like with Whole Grain Cereals you need to look for those breads that have as the first ingredient – Whole wheat, whole rye, whole oats, etc. And like it was discussed in Secret #58 your bread must have more fiber than sugar. This seems like it would be easy but it is not.

More Fiber than Sugar."

With bread there is another ingredient that you must watch out for and that is Sodium or Salt! Try to stay under 200 mg per slice. We get enough salt in all our other foods so keep it down on the breads.

Here are the numbers for the bread that I buy from the local grocery store – Great Grains Bakery, Multigrain Flax Seeds & Omerga-3. It may not be the best on the market but it is affordable and the numbers look good:

Per Slice - serving
- Sodium – 170 mg
- Total Carbohydrates – 24 grams
- Dietary Fiber – 5 grams
- Sugars – 1 grams
- Protein – 5 grams

The sodium is low and there is more fiber and protein than most bread and the sugar is low. But like anything else, keep the consumption of the bread down even if it is healthy, moderation in all things.

If you have gluten intolerance then you will have to look for a healthy alternative.

> **ACTION ITEM: If you can eat bread and tolerate whole grains, this week look and try to upgrade the quality of your breads to more whole grains. Just make sure there is more fiber than sugar and it will be an improvement over the standard white bread.**

60. VEGETABLES - 5-7 Servings Daily

The serving sizes vary but as a general rule ½ cup of chopped, cooked or raw veggies is considered 1 serving. When it comes to raw leafy vegetables like a green salad, a serving is 1 cup. Since different vegetables contain different amounts of nutrients eat a variety.

As bare minimum, eat dark green leafy vegetables such as kale, spinach and beet greens several times a week. These are really loaded with vitamins and minerals. These are easy to put into your diet. Just put them in a salad instead of, or in addition to, the iceberg lettuce.

Unless you are a vegetarian or vegan you probably are not in the habit of eating a lot of vegetables. So what will it take for you to get into the habit of eating 5-7 servings of vegetables each day? Here are a few tips.

a. Constantly remind yourself to eat more veggies, even if you need to put post-it notes up.
b. Have veggies available everywhere: home, work and eating out.
c. Make it easy and quick for you and your family.
d. Start to add the veggies in slowly over a couple of weeks. This will allow your body to adjust. Veggies contain lots of fiber.

Here are a couple of ideas on how to get more vegetables into your daily diet.

a. Throw some veggies into a skillet and then add in a couple of eggs.
b. Eat a dark leafy green salad most days and add in different veggies such as carrots, zucchini, broccoli and cucumbers to beef it up.
c. Add some vegetables into some of your favorite dishes like zucchini into your lasagna, broccoli spears into the mac and cheese or your quesadillas. You get the idea.
d. Have a good hearty vegetable soup once a week and a nice vegetable stew.

You will definitely notice a difference in your health and moods when you increase the amount of vegetables in your daily diet.

ACTION ITEM: This week increase the amount of veggies in your daily meals and see how you feel at the end of the week.

61. THE GREAT EXPERIMENT: Vegetable And Fruit Smoothies

Since the USDA's recommendation is 5-7 servings of vegetables and 2-3 servings of fruit a day, a great way to get this amount into your daily diet is through smoothies and especially green smoothies. There are hundreds if not thousands of green smoothie recipes available to you on the internet. (See the links below for some recipes)

Smoothies and Juices are NOT the same thing. Juicing takes everything out (pulp) except the juice. Smoothies use most of the whole fruit or vegetable. Smoothies are usually loaded with fiber and other nutrients found in the pulp. So I prefer smoothies over juices.

If you are new to making and drinking smoothies here are a couple of beginner tips;

- In the beginning, use more fruit than dark leafy greens and other veggies.
- Over a few weeks, slowly add in more veggies and less fruit.
- Once your smoothies are a majority of veggies you can experiment with the 'other greens' like green algae chlorophyll, alfalfa sprouts, etc., as they have very strong flavors. Start with just a sprinkle and work up.
- You can try adding in protein powders or foods that are high in protein like chia seeds or ground flax seeds.
- Make sure you have a high quality blender. Cheap blenders may leave chunks and not make the drink smooth.

Again, experiment and see what works best for you. Try different recipes and find a few that you like the best and start using them in your daily meal plans. I drink smoothies every week day morning for breakfast and save the heavier breakfasts for the weekend.

ACTION ITEM: This week find two smoothie recipes and try them out. Then keep trying different recipes until you have 5-6 that you really like and add them into your daily diet.

Smoothie Recipes:
http://healthyblenderrecipes.com/recipes/raw_vegan_spicy_veget able_green_smoothie

http://www.incrediblesmoothies.com/recipes/big-blend-fruit-vegetable-smoothie-recipe/

62. WHOLE FOODS - RICH IN ANTIOXIDANTS - BERRIES IN SEASON

Berries are special because they contain high levels of phytochemicals, which help protect cells from free radical damage. It is the damage by free radicals that cause aging, disease and all other physical problems with the body.

Eating berries has a huge impact on the brain and improves memory and helps elevate moods. According to research, berries contain 'Polyphenolics' which helps in the cleaning process in the brain and helps remove toxins and build-up of toxins from the brain. This helps the brain function properly and helps with memory retention.

In another study the researchers found that women who ate two servings of strawberries or one serving of blueberries a week showed less mental decline than those women who did not eat berries during the study. This is due to a group of compounds called 'Anthocyanidins'. These compounds are able to cross the blood-brain barrier and get in to the brain to work their magic.

Here is a list of some of the antioxidants that are found in berries.

- Anthocyanins
- Quercetin
- Vitamin C
- Polyphenolics

These are powerful antioxidants that have a wide variety of positive effects on the brain and body such as reducing inflammation in the body. Pesticides and herbicides are routinely used in the production of berries and especially blueberries, so use organic berries when possible.

If you feel physically healthy you will be more inclined to feel mentally healthy.

ACTION ITEM: This week add a couple of servings of fresh berries into your meal plan. Blueberries are a wonderful addition to Buckwheat pancakes. Strawberries and Blackberries are great in smoothies.

63. HEALTHY SNACKS - Create A Daily Snack Plate

The idea here is to have your healthy snacks prepared in advance and easily available when that 'Snack Attack' hits.

I can remember years ago, as a child, visiting my grandparent's farm and seeing a big bowl of fruit on the counter. If I was hungry, and it was not close to meal time, I knew I could just grab an apple or banana and eat it. It was quick, easy and I did not have to ask.

You can do the same thing but with a slight twist – Include Vegetables. Make a plate with fruit and veggies on it and set it out. Then throughout the day when you (or a family member) are hungry you can just grab a carrot stick or slices of zucchini – you get the idea. You can also put some nuts and seeds there also.

On work days you can have snack bags pre-prepared, full of fruit slices, veggies, nuts or seeds. You can just grab one and throw it in with your lunch and take it with you. If you don't have it with you at work you are going to run to the vending machine and buy junk food.

Nearly every morning I put my snack bags together. I have one small snack bag full of veggie slices, such as carrots, sweet potato, small sweet peppers and zucchini. The other snack bag is full of homemade granola or a mixture of dried fruit, nuts and seeds and I alternate throughout the week.

This is a simple idea, to prepare your healthy snacks ahead of time, and have them available when the need arises. It does not take long to put a healthy snack plate together and the rewards are great. You must feed your body healthy snacks if you want the brain to be healthy and to have a healthy and happy life.

ACTION ITEM: Every day this week make a healthy snack plate if you or your family is going to be home. On work days take a healthy snack bag with you to enjoy at work.

64. VITAMIN L - LOVE In Home Cooking

One of the most potent vitamins found in some foods, one which can kill cancer cells, reduce pain and improve mental health is Vitamin L – LOVE!

Which foods contain the most Vitamin L? Answer: Most all Home Cooked Meals contain generous portions. Cooking meals at home is how the love gets in the food. If the food is 'home-grown' it even contains more Vitamin L.

Think back to when you were growing up. It always seems like grandma's cooking tasted so good. Everyone could hardly wait until meal time to see what grandma had cooked up. It was because grandma put so much of her time, effort and love into the meals.

Another example – I can remember how much better peanut-- butter and jam sandwiches tasted when my mother made them for me. They always tasted better than the ones I made myself, even though I used the same peanut butter and jam. It was because my mother put some of her love into making the sandwich.

Vitamin L can be obtained from eating home cooked meals together, as a family, around the dinner table. Love and food have been known to be 'the glue' that holds families together. Traditions are born and preserved around the dinner table eating home cooked meals.

Even if you are single and eat alone, cook your meals from scratch, using whole foods, and put a little care and thought into the meal. You can feed yourself a little – self-love.

ACTION ITEM: This week eat at home, around the table as a family, while enjoying meals cooked from scratch. Make sure you put thought and love into the food while preparing the meal.

65. HEALTHY, TRADITIONAL FATS – Butter, Olive Oil and Coconut Oil

"Eat Healthy Fats!"
"Eating Healthy Fats Does Not Make You Fat!"

For the last several decades you have been told to eat a 'low fat' diet. All the dietitians, doctors and such said that eating too much fat was bad for the heart and made you fat. Well in recent years, studies are showing that this is not necessarily true. It all depends on which types of fats you eat. There are some very healthy fats that you don't have to really worry about eating too much.

You should be getting 20%-35% of your calories from healthy fats according to the 2010 Dietary Guideline for Americans.

Just make sure that most of your fats come from the following sources...

Coconut Oil: This oil is loaded with medium-chain fatty acids. These are much easier for your body to digest and harder for the body to store as fat. Also these are broken down into smaller sizes so the cells can utilize the energy almost immediately. Coconut Oil is gaining a reputation for improving memory and brain functions.

Real Butter: Butter nearly became a casualty in the war on fat or the low-fat diet craze. Butter is now making a recovery since the health benefits of butter are becoming more widely accepted. Real Butter contains good healthy Omega-3 and Omega-6 which are known to help improve skin health and especially important for healthy brain functions.

Extra Virgin Olive Oil (EVOO): Several cultures have known about the health benefits of EVOO for centuries. All diets should include Olive Oil. This oil contains high amounts of antioxidants which protects all your cells from damage. As with the previous mentioned healthy oils, EVOO is great for memory and cognitive function plus it reduces inflammation.

Non-Traditional Sources of healthy fats

Avocado – These are one of the healthiest fruits you can eat because of the numerous health benefits. This delicious green treat is rich in monounsaturated fats, which lower the bad cholesterol while raising the good cholesterol. The Avocado is loaded with Vitamin E and Vitamin E is great at preventing free radical damage and helps boost your immune system.

Don't forget that the Avocado is loaded with healthy protein and has more than any other fruit.

Omega-3 Fatty Acids: Since our bodies cannot produce Omega-3's we must rely on our diet to supply these nutrients. There are 3 different kinds or types of Ogema-3s: EPA – eicosapetaenoic acid, DHA – docosahexaenoic acid and ALA – alpha-linolenic acid. The one's you need to be the most concerned with is EPA and DHA. They are found in sea-foods like Salmon and Sardines. ALA is found in some plant foods, most notably, nuts and seeds and in high quality grass-fed beef.

Include Fats in your daily diet. Don't be afraid that you will gain a ton of weight because it just won't happen. I use lots of coconut oil in cooking my vegetables, put avocados in my smoothies and butter on my buckwheat pancakes. I am staying slim and trim and feel great. So can you.

ACTION ITEM: This week start incorporating more healthy fats like Avocado, Coconut Oil and Olive Oil into your meals. Your brain, body and mood will thank you.

66. REFINED SEED AND VEGETABLE OILS - Cut and Reduce

There are good fats and bad fats. In secret number 65 we talked about how to add healthy fats into your diet. Well now we are going to talk about the unhealthy fats that you need to remove from your diet.

Not all fats and oils are created equal. Many oils are unhealthy and hazardous to your health. These oils are highly processed and heated, cleaned with chemicals and use GMO corn, canola or soy.

Do a google search and watch a couple of video's on how vegetable oil is made. It will change your mind about your cooking oils.

Here is a partial list of some of these oils that you should start to work on reducing from your diet and replacing with the healthy fats in #65.

- o Vegetable Oil
- o Soybean Oil
- o Corn Oil
- o Canola Oil
- o Hydrogenated Oils
- o Margarine
- o Any oil that is labeled as refined, hydrogenated, partially-hydrogenated

These oils contain huge amounts of Polyunsaturated fatty acids called Omega-6, which can be harmful to your cells if you consume to many. If the ratio of Omega-6 to Omega-3 is too high it can be harmful to your body and mind. Your ratio needs to be in the 4:1 to 1:2 ranges. The average American diet has a ration as high as 16:1. This is why you need to either increase your Omega-3 fatty acids and/or reduce the Omega-6 fatty acids. The best plan of attack is to do both – reduce the Omega-6 and increase the Omega-3 in your daily diet.

These types of oils contribute to inflammation, loaded with trans fats, increase your risk of heart disease and ratio of Omega -6 to Omega -3 has been shown to have a strong association with risk of severe depression.

So for better overall health and to lower your risk of depression work on getting as many of these highly processed oils out of your diet. Your body and mind will love you for it.

***ACTION ITEM: To help improve you moods and
overall health start to remove and replace these
unhealthy seed and vegetable oils with the healthy
coconut oil, olive oil and avocados.***

67. MIDDAY SUNSHINE - VITAMIN D, The Missing Nutritional Link

It is estimated that more than 1 billion people worldwide are deficient in vitamin D. Why is this true? Answer: Humans are spending less time in the sun today than at any point in human history.

One of the most important preventive measures you can take to improve your overall health and happiness is to make sure you get sufficient amounts of Vitamin D. <u>There are now hundreds of studies that link Vitamin D deficiency to higher risk of many different cancers, heart disease, and depression.</u>

Signs of Deficiency:

1. You Feel Blue – Studies indicate that those with the lowest levels of vitamin D were 11 times more at risk to be depressed than those who received healthy daily doses.
2. Bones Ache / Soft Bones - Aches and Pains and Fatigue.
3. Cognitive impairment in older adults.
4. Increase death rate from cardiovascular disease.

The best source and the only natural source of Vitamin D is SUNLIGHT. When you get your Vitamin D from sunshine your body uses only what it needs and gets rid of the extra. If you are deficient you will need 2,000 – 5,000 IU a day. But if you are in the normal range you will need 1,000 – 2,000 IU a day.

Here is list of several good sources and quantities of Vitamin D you can expect to get from them.

Sunlight Exposure   10-15 minutes (arms and legs exposure v.s. most of the body exposed – Depending on where on the earth you are living)   3,000 – 20,000 IU

Salmon (3.5 oz. of fresh, wild caught)   600 - 1,000 IU
Salmon (3.5 oz. of fresh, farmed raised)   100 – 250 IU
Milk, Fortified (8 oz. glass) (milk has no natural Vitamin D) 100 IUA

As you can see Sunshine is the best source, if you live where there is strong enough, and enough quantity of UVB rays to provide Vitamin D. So here is my recommendation, unless you live within a thousand miles from the Equator – go on a 15 minute walk around noon and take a Vitamin D supplement.

Get your daily dose of vitamin D – first from the sunshine and second from supplementation. Either way, make sure you are getting enough of this Sunshine Vitamin for a healthy mind, body and overall great health. So when you are feeling 'blue' increase your daytime walking.

ACTION ITEM: Don't rely on drinking a glass of milk for your dose of Vitamin D. Increase your day time walking AND take a good quality Vitamin D supplement and watch your spirit soar.

68.   FIRMENTED FOODS - Health Starts In The Gut

A healthy gut is the keystone to having a healthy body and mind. If you have a leaky gut or your gut bacteria are all out of balance, your body will feel lousy and your mind and moods can be way out of balance.

There are a lot of different nutritional therapies that can help improve your health but one that can really boost your overall health and wellness is adding fermented foods to your diet. Your gut needs help to heal and become healthy and eating different fermented foods is just the answer.

All the different fermented foods are just over-flowing with good bacteria or 'probiotics'. There are also countless research studies demonstrating how having a balance of good and bad bacteria in your gut forms the foundation for mental, emotional, physical and overall wellbeing.

Here are some benefits of eating traditional, fermented foods;

- *Loaded With Important Nutrients* – Some fermented foods are a great source of Vitamin K2. Just 15 grams of Natto daily provide all your daily K2 needs. B Vitamins are plentiful in fermented food.
- *Body Detoxification* – The beneficial bacteria are great detoxers (if this is a real word). They are capable of withdrawing a wide range of different heavy metals and toxins from the body. Fermented foods are great chelators which aid in detoxification.
- *Natural Source and Variety Of Microflora* – Supplements only contain a few different beneficial bacteria but eating a

variety of fermented foods will add a much wider array of beneficial bacteria into your gut.

- *Boosting Your Immune System* – Did you know that your gut contains around 80% of your immune system? Probiotics and a healthy gut play a critical role in the development and the operation of the mucosal immune system in your digestive tract. And this aids in the production of antibodies to kill pathogens.
- *Cost Effective* – Adding small amounts of good quality or homemade fermented foods to each of your meals will give you 100 times more probiotics than most supplements.

Here is a short list of fermented foods (buy at health food store when possible);

- Tempeh (fermented soybeans)
- Miso (fermented paste made from barley, rice or soybeans)
- Sauerkraut - Raw (fermented cabbage – easy to make at home)
- Yogurt (labeled – "Live & Active Cultures")
- Kefer (fermented milk drink – easy to make at home)
- Kombucha (fermented tea – can be made at home)
- Kimchi (Korean fermented cabbage)
- Other Misc. Vegetables

You must have good gut health if you want to achieve a higher level of over-all wellness and improved moods. To obtain and maintain good gut health you need to add fermented foods to your daily diet or take a probiotic supplement. Check out the GAP diet if you really need to heal your digestive system. Probiotic foods are an important part of this diet. It is a great diet for Autism and most mood disorders.

ACTION ITEM: This week add some real, unpasteurized fermented foods into your daily diet. Go slow with small amounts and build up from there. Alternative: Start taking a high quality probiotic supplement to start improving your gut health.

69.   EGGS: Buy Quality - The Healthy Protein

Eggs are among some of the most nutritious foods as they contain a little bit of almost every nutrient your body needs to maintain wellness. The whole egg contains all the required nutrients to turn a single cell into a baby chicken.

Try to buy quality and purchase either Omega-3 enriched or pastured/free ranged eggs. These even contain a lot more Omega-3's and Vitamin A and E than the cheaper eggs. It is worth the investment.

A single egg is packed with 77 calories, **6 grams of high quality protein** and 5 grams of healthy fats. The quality of the protein is so high Eggs are used as the standard by which all other foods are measured. Remember Rocky Balboa (Sylvester Stallone) chugging down those drinks full of raw eggs as he trained for the big fight? He needed the high quality protein to help build muscle, strength and endurance. (I don't recommend drinking raw eggs)

Eating a couple of eggs in the morning will give you enough fats and especially protein to keep you feeling full and give you the energy needed to keep going till lunch. Protein is needed throughout the day for good health.

Many people will not eat eggs out of fear that they will raise their blood cholesterol levels. It is true that eggs are high in cholesterol, BUT they do not affect blood cholesterol. The reason is – the liver actually produces large amounts of cholesterol every single day, so when you eat eggs, the liver just produces less cholesterol instead. So the cholesterol level remains consistent. Eating eggs will raise the "good" cholesterol (HDL) which is a good thing.

EXTRA BENEFIT - Eggs are a brain food! 1 whole egg contains 100 mg of CHOLINE. Several different dietary surveys show that nearly 90% of all the people in the U.S. are not getting the recommended daily amount of choline. In other words, most likely you are deficient in choline.

Choline is used to produce signaling molecules that are used in the brain. You may be wondering why your mind is not as sharp as it should be and why you may be suffering from depression, anxiety or some other mood disorder. It may be because you are deficient in Choline. Eat a couple of eggs and give your brain and mood a boost.

Eggs are healthy and they are not to be avoided unless of course you are on the vegan diet, or you have a known intolerance or allergy.

ACTION ITEM: This week try adding in a couple of extra eggs into your diet. If you already eat eggs on a regular basis, try upgrading the quality of the eggs and buy Free Range Eggs or at least the Omega-3 enriched eggs.

70. WHOLE GRAIN FLOURS - Use As Fresh As Possible

Nothing tastes better than fresh, homemade bread from freshly ground flour and other healthy ingredients. Let's not forget about the higher nutritional value of using fresh ingredients.

Whole grain flour loses most of it nutritional value within a few days of being ground. Also the wheat germ oil that is found in whole grain flour will start to turn rancid. So think about how long that whole grain flour has been sitting on the grocery store shelf before you end up buying it. This is one reason some flour smells a little rancid or moldy.

There is some testing that shows that within 72 hours of the milling or grinding process up to 90% of the nutritional value has been destroyed. Once most of the vitamin and minerals have been destroyed and the flour turns rancid the only thing left are some empty calories from mainly starch. When you eat starch it quickly turns to sugar which causes glucose spikes within the body.

If you buy freshly ground flour you will know that you are getting the most nutritional value possible. You will know that you are getting the whole grain and all the nutrients possible such as:

- Insoluble fiber,
- Magnesium
- Riboflavin
- Thiamine and Niacin
- Iron, Zinc
- Vitamins B1, B2, B3, E
- Polyunsaturated Fatty Acids

So when you want to bake, use only the freshest whole grain flour possible. Either grind your own or find a bakery or other retail outlet that grinds whole grains daily. Whole grains are an excellent source for fiber and other important ingredients. Your body and brain will appreciate you and reward you with awesome health and a more stable mind.

ACTION ITEM: This week find a retail outlet that sells fresh ground whole grain flour. Then get rid of all the white flour or old whole grain flour that you have in your kitchen.

71. CHIA SEEDS - King of Energy, Omega-3 Fatty Acids, Protein and Fiber

I Love Chia Seeds! I put these little seeds in my drinking water, which makes the water alkaline. I put them in my 'overnight refrigerator oatmeal' that I eat as part of my lunch. I even add them to my buckwheat pancakes. These little seeds are chuck full of great nutritional stuff.

Chia seeds are a great source of Omega-3 Fatty Acids, Protein and Fiber. They are a great source of Magnesium, Manganese, and Phosphorus, providing about 1/3 of our daily requirements with just 2 tablespoons a day.

Here a few other reasons to add Chia Seeds to your daily diet:

- Weight Loss – due to the high protein and fiber weight loss can be enhanced with chia seeds

- Loaded with Antioxidants – Helps to destroy free radicals that cause diseases
- Loaded with important bone health nutrients like calcium and magnesium
- Improves Exercise Performance – The Ancient Aztec warriors ate chia seeds especially before battles.
- Very easy to incorporate into your diet. They are rather tasteless so you can add them to most dishes without disturbing the favor.
- Lower in real carbohydrates – Most of the carbs in Chia Seeds come in the form of insoluble fiber.

Again I just love Chia Seeds and I know you will too. Start by adding some Chia seeds to your bottled water (gently shake the bottle for a minute or two first to keep from forming a glob on the bottom) and you will notice a difference. Give your body the nutrients it needs to keep itself healthy.

ACTION ITEM: Purchase some Chia Seeds and start adding some to your water, sprinkle on yogurt or add some to your pancakes or other baked goods.

72. DEEP FRIED FOODS - Know The Oil Used!

Before you eat any foods that are deep fried find out what oil(s) were used. Many restaurants and fast food establishments cook their fried foods using man made oils that contain trans fats. These trans fats can be reused over and over again which helps keep the cost down for the establishment. Partially Hydrogenated Oils contains trans fats and is another name some people use instead of trans fats.

According to the American Heart Association – Trans Fats (partially hydrogenated oil) can 'lead to heart disease' in some people. The evidence is quite convincing. So much so that several European countries and Canada have either banned trans fats or severely restrict its use.

Many of these different vegetable oils and trans fats are created in an industrial chemical making process that adds hydrogen to a liquid vegetable oil to make them more solid when not heated. The main source for these trans fats are found in processed food with an ingredient called "partially hydrogenated oils".

Back in November of 2013, the FDA put out a statement that said partially hydrogenated oils were no longer classified as 'Generally Recognized As Safe' in foods for humans. The main reason companies put these fats into their processed foods is because it gives foods a desirable texture as well as flavor.

Here are 3 types of oils you should remove from your deep fried cooking.

1. Canola Oil – It comes from one of the top 3 GMO foods in the U.S. and is used by most all restaurants and fried foods in the grocery stores.
2. Corn Oil / Corn by-products - Again this is a GMO based oil and foods. The GMO contains pesticides to protect again bugs. When you eat this you potentially are putting these pesticides into your body.
3. Soy based Oils and Soy by-products – All soybeans are now GMO unless specified otherwise.

There is only a couple of ways that you can eliminate or reduce your exposure to trans fats. One - before you order your meal at a restaurant or a fast food establishment, ask which oil they use. Two - before buying fried foods look at the label to see what oil was used. Just by removing most fried foods from your diet will go a long way toward losing weight, and improving your overall health. Another healthy tip: Replace the trans fats in your diet with monounsaturated or polyunsaturated fats, these are the healthy types of fats.

ACTION ITEM: This week find out what oils are being use to cook your foods. Try to reduce the amount of fried food you eat, especially if it is cooked with Trans-fat oils.

73.   LIFE'S BEST HEALTH LESSON: Plant A Vegetable Garden

Gardening is one of my hobbies. It is a place where I can come home from work and relax as I plant, water and harvest. I have a couple of small fruit trees on one end of the garden space. I have blueberries, raspberries and my pride and joy – Goji berries. I have a Strawberry patch and 5-6 raised beds where I grow different types of squash, kale, tomatoes, beans, etc.

You may even have done some gardening in the past. So here is a question to think about – 'Why do a garden'? My answer may surprise you – "*It is the best health lesson*". I find peace and relaxation and for a little while the cares and worries of life are left outside the garden. Everyone needs a place where they can do some deep thinking. Mine is while I am digging in the dirt prepping the soil. I think about my life – the good times, the trials and what I have learned from them.

I don't consider working in my garden work – well except on those hot July and August evenings when I water the garden. I just enjoy being outdoors and listening to the birds and a couple of chattering squirrels in the nearby trees. Another great reward is bringing in and eating the harvest.

You and your Family can have a similar experience by putting in a small garden in the corner of the back yard. Here is another advantage – your kids will eat more vegetables if they helped to plant, water and pick them. Home grown veggies and fruit are the healthiest foods you can eat.

Gardens provide some pretty good exercise also. Gardens teach you and your children about 'The Law Of The Harvest' – you reap what you sow. Gardens will teach your children reverence and greater appreciation for the food they eat when they help grow it.

Yes, there are many lessons on health that can be learned or accomplished by growing a garden. While your garden is growing you and your family will learn some pretty important health lessons, if you will just take the time to look for them.

Even if you live in an apartment you can grow a few simple vegetables or herbs in potted containers. In some areas there are community gardens that you can get involved with and enjoy working together to grow food. Your spirits will soar as you put work and love into growing food.

ACTION ITEM: This week evaluate your situation and see if you can grow a garden. If so plan it out and start working toward having your own garden.

74. EAT A RAINBOW - Colors Of Fruits And Vegetables Matter!

Try eating all the different colors when it comes to fruits and vegetables. Think – red, dark green, yellow, white, orange, blue and purple. This will provide your dishes with eye appealing color but more importantly – a broad range of nutrients. So 'think variety, think color' and you and your family can win the healthy nutrition game.

When you eat a variety of colors you know that you are getting as many of the different vitamin and minerals as possible. Make sure you are getting a wide variety of foods within each color. You must get a variety of foods in order to get all the needed vitamins, minerals and essential nutrients your body needs to be healthy and happy. This is especially true if you are a 'picky' eater.

The Color Key for Fruits and Vegetables:

Yellow and Orange – Vitamins C and A (Citrus Fruits, Squash)

Green – Vitamins K, B and E (Avocado, Kale, Spinach)

Purple – Vitamins C and K (Grapes, Eggplant, Red Cabbage)

You get the idea. The plants get their colors from the different phytochemicals found in them. It is these different phytochemicals or colors that offer the different nutrients when they are eaten.

When it comes to your overall health and mood enhancement, just remember that focusing on just one vitamin or nutrient is generally a bad idea. You will do more good by just eating a well-balanced and well-rounded diet and you will get most of the nutrients you need, in a form that your body will be able to use.

It might be a dumb saying – 'Eat the Rainbow' but it comes with a lot of wisdom and experience. So for your physical and mental health – "Eat The Rainbow" – add variety and color to your diet and your body and mind will be healthier and happier.

ACTION ITEM: This week eat some different fruits and vegetables that you may not have eaten before or in a long time. Add variety and color to your daily diet.

75. OLD FASHION VITAMINS – Whole Foods (Veggies, Fruit, Legumes, Nuts, Whole Grains And A Little Meat

How did your Grandparents or Great Grandparents get their daily dose of daily vitamins and minerals?

It was one of two sources: Cod Liver Oil (if the family could afford it) and Whole Foods.

Getting your vitamins from Whole Foods is a novel idea. Your grandparents did not have all the supplement pills we have today. They had to get most everything from whole foods like – Veggies, Fruit, Legumes, Nuts, Whole Grains and a little Meat.

When you were little and went to visit your grandparents or great grandparents, what do you remember eating? I remember home cooked meals – home made everything. The soups were generally homemade, along with the bread. The meals always

143

seemed to have a little of everything, veggies, beans, nuts whole grains and some meat.

Today, the prevailing attitude is – Eat what you want and take a cheap 1 A-Day Vitamin and all is well. Your grandparents believed in eating nutritious whole food meals and then take a spoonful of good quality Cod Liver Oil just in case.

So for good health, a healthy mind and happiness, take a stroll down memory lane and return to your roots and cook some of your grandma's traditional whole food meals. It will warm your heart and soul, not to mention improves your mood. Get some of those important old fashion vitamins into your daily diet.

ACTION ITEM: Get a few of your grandparent's favorite recipes that were handed down and try them this week. For an extra treat get their favorite stew or soup recipes.

76. SUPPLEMENTS: A Time And Place (Omega-3, Vitamin D and Probiotics)

The time and place is today. IF you are eating a well-balanced whole food diet you may not need to supplement your vitamin and mineral needs. Let's assume you are one of the few people who take your lifestyle diet serious, you still may need to take supplements in three key nutrients. I highly recommend supplements for these three key nutrients:

- **Omega-3 Fatty Acids – Fish Oils**. Why? Because you would have to eat a lot of wild caught salmon to get enough Omega-3's to counter-balance the excessive amounts of Omega-6's in the Standard American Diet. Too much Omega-6's cause inflammation. Omega-3's fight off inflammation in the body.
- **Vitamin D** – As you may know most people in the United State live way north of the Equator plus we seem to be too afraid to go outside in the sun. Being in the sunlight is the only natural way of getting vitamin D. Some people drink milk to get vitamin D but you would have to drink gallons of milk a day to get the amount your body needs.
- **Probiotics** – If you are not eating a well-balanced diet with sufficient amounts of different fiber you probably have gut issues. The other alternative is to eat different fermented foods like fresh non-cooked or pasteurized sauerkraut. Most people do not like nor eat much fermented foods. So to get or maintain a healthy gut you must be feeding the microbiome within the gut.

So at a minimum, if you are eating the standard diet of highly processed foods, you must supplement in those three areas. If you do, make sure that the supplements are high quality. If so you will feel a difference. Depression / anxiety symptoms can be caused by a poor diet and a deficiency in key vitamins and minerals. So if you want to have a healthy body and mind consider taking supplements in these three key areas.

ACTION ITEMS: This week pick up some high quality Vitamin D, Fish Oil and Probiotics and plan on taking them for 90 days and see how you feel. You will be pleasantly surprised with the results.

77. PROTEIN: Eat Twice As Much Plant Protein Than Animal Protein

There is a huge debate in the world of nutrition concerning eating meat and how much meat a person should eat. We need protein in order to build muscle, rebuild cells and just plain be healthy. Meat is not the only source of protein, unless you have gluten intolerance.

There are several reasons that you should get the bulk of your protein from plant sources. Each source of protein has its advantages and disadvantages.

- Meat Protein:
    - Advantage – Complete source of all amino acids including all essential amino acids. Rich source of zinc and Iron (easier to absorb by the body than Iron from plant-based foods.)
    - Disadvantage – Can contain higher levels of saturated fats and dietary cholesterol. Contains low levels of fiber. The body has a harder time getting rid of excess meat proteins. Unless you get organic meat (can be hard to find and expensive) you expose your body to anti-biotics, growth hormones, etc.
- Plant Protein:
    - Advantage – Lower intake of dietary cholesterol and unhealthy saturated fats. Easier to find Organic plant proteins than Organic meats. You have to eat a variety of plant proteins to get ALL non-essential amino acids – thus getting a wider range of other valuable vitamins and minerals. Eating plant protein

will also give you lots of fiber (you get two great nutrients for eating one source). The body can get rid of extra plant protein easier than meat protein.

  o Disadvantage – Soy Protein contains isoflavones, which resembles the female hormone – Estrogen. Too much estrogen in some women causes weight gain and a host of other unwanted health issues. You have to eat a variety of plant protein to get all the essential proteins. (But I listed it as an advantage also.)

Because of the advantages and disadvantages listed above, I recommend eating twice as much plant based protein than meat protein. There is also one more overall advantage of eating more plant protein than meat protein – According to a 2010 review of numerous studies, an article was published in "Nutrition in Clinical Practice" stated that individuals following vegetarian type diets have <u>lower body mass indexes,</u> <u>lower blood cholesterol</u> levels and <u>lower blood pressure </u>than non-vegetarians.

Adapt this secret into your daily diet and see if you don't feel better, have happier moods and overall sense of wellness.

ACTION ITEM: This next week or two try eating less meat and more plant based proteins, such as, Quinoa, Soy (Tofu, Tempeh), legumes and other whole grains.

78. KALE AND SWISS CHARD: Eat A Dark Leafy Green Salad Every Day

Have you heard the saying; *'A Large Dark Leafy Green Salad A Day Keeps The Doctors Away?'* You haven't!! Well it's true! Dark Leafy Greens are the king of the veggies and Kale just might be the greatest of them all.

Here is just a small list of the healthy benefits of Kale and some of the other dark leafy greens.

- o Vitamin K – Just one cup of raw kale or any of the other dark leafy greens will give you adequate amounts of vitamin K. Deficiency in Vitamin K can lead to kidney and artery calcification, weak bones and cardiovascular disease. More info on Vitamin K in tip #84.
- o Lowers Cholesterol – Kale and Mustard Greens lower cholesterol. Steamed seems to work better for this. The fiber in these greens combines with bile to remove cholesterol.
- o Prevents Eye Damage – Spinach, Kale, Swiss Chard along with a number of other dark leafy greens contains a lot of carotenoids, zeaxanthin and lutein. These nutrients help filter high-energy light that can cause eye damage.
- o High Calcium – Mustard Greens contains 55 mg; Swiss Chard contains 54 mg; and Kale has 49 mg. The slightly bitter taste reflects the higher levels of calcium.
- o Reduction In Risk For Colon Cancer – Kale, Cabbage, Broccoli and Mustard Greens helped reduce the risk of colon cancer in a 2011 study published in the Journal of the American Dietetic Association.

For better health, whip up and eat a Caesar salad, or any other dark leafy green salad, every day. So as you can see – 'A Salad A Day Can Keep The Doctors Away!"

HINT: Use a healthy Oil and Vinegar salad dressing instead of the unhealthy creamy type dressings.

ACTION ITEM: Every day this week, eat a big dark leafy green salad, with healthier Vinegar and Oil based salad dressing. This is not a salad made up of a lot of iceberg lettuce and a few shredded carrots. This is salad with kale, spinach, chard and a host of other dark leafy greens and veggies.

79. FASTING: The Monthly Detox

There is an age-old religious practice that has some real health benefits - Fasting. There is one faith in particular that has fasting as part of their regular religious practices. The Church of Jesus Christ of Latter-day Saints (Mormons) practice a 24 hour fast, usually on the first Sunday of each month.

Some initial studies have shown that there are health benefits to fasting. One study showed a correlation between fasting and reduction in the risk of developing diabetes. Another study showed a lower rate of heart disease among those that practice regular fasting – at least once a month.

But one of the main benefits of doing a 24 hour fast is it gives the body and its organs, such as your digestive system a chance to rest. Fasting may not provide a significant time to detox but it gives the detoxing organs a little rest. It also allows the body to burn up any extra glucose in your blood stream. Because of this, diabetics may not be able to fast for as long or may need to do a juice fast instead.

There are some health benefits of fasting but there are other benefits as well. Members of The Church of Jesus Christ of Latter-day Saints are encouraged to donate the value of the two meals that they missed as a 'fast offering' to help provide for those who may be less fortunate or poor. They also believe that there is a spiritual component also – bringing their spirit closer to God as they pray during this time – usually for someone else who is struggling in life. So while you give your body a time to rest, you can be giving a chance for your spirit to grow. Your body will feel rested and rejuvinated after the fast. Your mind will be a little less foggy.

ACTION ITEM: Try 'Fasting' one day this month by going without food and water. If you have medical conditions then drink some juice throughout the day.

80.   DAIRY: Use It Sparingly

Did you know that up to 75% of the people of the world have either a lactose or casein intolerance or allergy? 90% of African American's and 80% of the Asians are lactose intolerant. These numbers are the results of thousands of studies.

Lactose and Casein are both found in milk. If you take the time to think about it you would come to realize that humans are the only species that deliberately drink the milk of another animal. Do you normally see a pig sucking on a cow or a puppy sucking on a sheep? You get the point. Is it natural or healthy in the long run? This is just something to think about.

So if this is true it should not be any surprise to find out that your immune system may not recognize milk and its proteins and sugars as friendly food.

Lactose Intolerance just means you do not have the ability to digest Lactose, which is a sugar in milk. Since there is a huge brain-gut connection, when the gut is irritated by a food it can send bad signals to the brain. In one study, subjects who had lactose intolerance showed a significantly higher score on the Beck depression inventory test, compared to those without the lactose intolerance. Other symptoms include-

- Gas and Bloating
- Loose Stools or Diarrhea
- Throwing Up or Nausea
- Depression Like Symptoms

Casein allergy or intolerance is when the body thinks this dairy protein is a foreign invader. This attack on the casein protein causes the body many different problems. This type of intolerance or allergy is harder to diagnose and takes longer for the symptoms to appear. These symptoms may be;

- Diarrhea or chronic Constipation
- Foggy Brain or Tingly Fingers and hands
- Joint Pain or Symptoms of Depression / Anxiety

The symptom of these two dairy intolerances can be very similar but then again they can be very different. But the one thing they have in common is the cure or the solution. The solution is to remove milk and other dairy products from your diet.

If you are suffering from depression, anxiety or other mood disorders try removing dairy from your diet or minimize the amount you eat. It might just be as simple as a cure for your mood swings. You might find other benefits as well, such as less mucus and stuffy noses, less ear infections, etc.

ACTION ITEM: For 10 days remove all dairy from your diet and see what symptoms disappear. After 10 days slowly add dairy back into your diet and see if you notice any difference. You might be surprised to see your moods improve while you are off the dairy.

81. QUINOA, KASHA (BUCKWHEAT) AND OTHER WHOLE GRAINS

Eating whole grains is another area that is widely debated. The discussions all center on gluten and gluten intolerances. If you have sensitivity to gluten then by all means stay away from gluten containing grains. BUT if not then add healthy grains to your diet. They are packed with healthy nutrients that will feed the body and the brain. Here are a few grains/seeds that you might not have in your current diet that you might want to try. Some of these are gluten free.

QUINOA – (keen-wa)
- Gluten-Free
- Complete plant based Protein that includes all nine essential amino acids
- Contains high amounts of protein, fiber, magnesium, Iron and Omega-3 fatty acids

- Great replacement for pasta, rice or couscous which contain gluten

KASHA or BUCKWHEAT
- Gluten-Free
- High in minerals – magnesium, copper, manganese, phosphorus
- High Fiber contents
- Another good replacement for pasta or rice

SPELT
- The Nutrients are easily absorbed by the body because it is highly water soluble.
- Is much easier to digest than wheat and other grains because of its fragile gluten and high fiber content
- Good grain for those with digestive issues such as irritable bowel syndrome (IBS)
- Helps reduce LDL cholesterol levels and overall cholesterol levels
- Excellent source of phytoestrogens and lignans

MILLET
- Provides the body and brain Serotonin to help calm and level your moods
- Is Alkaline and Digests easily
- Is a prebiotic or a food for the microflora in your gut
- Is NOT a food for Candida
- Helps with having regular bowel movements because it hydrates your colon

As you can see, these different grains (some are technically seeds but used as grains) have different health benefits. It is important to have variety in your diet so as to get the different nutrients your body needs. It is true with grains/seeds, so eat a variety of these grains and notice how your body and mind feels. I think you will be pleasantly surprised.

ACTION ITEM: This week pick one or two of these grains/seeds and learn how to add them into your diet. You might have to go to a health food store to buy some of them. Your body and mind will thank you for it.

82. FAST FOODS - Eat The Healthiest Items - The Businesses Will Change

Only buy healthy items on the menu. These fast food places will never change unless we as consumers demand that they change. You do that by voting with your dollars. Here is just one example of an unhealthy meal – The World Famous McDonalds Big Mac

Big Mac   550 Calories   (This is just for the Big Mac – no fries, drink or cookie)

Nutrition Facts

Serving Size 1 sandwich (216 g)

Calories – 550	**Calories from Fat** - 261
Total Fat - 29g	**Saturated Fat** - 10g
Cholesterol - 75mg	**Sodium** - 970mg
Potassium - 0mg	**Carbohydrates** - 46g

Dietary Fiber - 3g   **Sugars** - 9g

Protein - 25g

Fast Food companies will not make many changes to their menus unless people stop buying these calorie loaded foods. So here is the fast food health tip of the day – Limit your fast food meals to 1 a week! Your mind, mood and body will really appreciate it and they will reward you for your restraint.

ACTION ITEM: Cut your intake of fast foods to just 1 meal a week and when you do buy, make the healthiest choice possible.

83. COLLECT HEALTHY TRADITIONAL FAMILY RECIPES

There is something special when you cook using recipes handed down from your mother or grandmother. Remember that dinner your mother cooked on special occasions that you just loved. Get the recipe before it is too late. But make sure they are the healthy ones, try to stay away from the cookies, and cake recipes since you are now trying to eat healthier.

I read a blog post from a gentleman whose father used to make the best homemade bread that he just loved. After his father passed away they could not find his special bread recipe anywhere. They later found out he made it from memory. Oh how this gentleman wished he had gotten that recipe from his father before his passing. Don't you wait until it is too late, get with your mother, grandmother, aunt or uncle and get their special recipes.

When you collect and use the healthy "traditional family" recipes you will help preserve some of the family traditions. This is especially true if the recipes originated from the 'mother' country. Since I am of German/Swiss descent, I sure wish I had my great grandmother's recipe for sauerkraut instead of the one I now use from off the internet.

There are several different ways you can save these recipes. Some individuals will start a Recipe Journal, either in a binder or on the computer. You can write them on recipe cards and file them the old fashion way, in a recipe box. Again it does not matter how you collect them, just start collecting them.

The other nice side benefit from doing this is it will give you an opportunity to visit with family members that you might not have visited with for a while. You can accomplish two things while trying to track down grandma's special apple pie recipe that you remembered eating as a child. It will give you a chance to walk down memory lane.

Your heart will be filled with fond memories as you cook from an old family recipe and your body and mind will be nourished in several different ways.

ACTION ITEM: This week contact your mother or grandmother and get at least 1 recipe of your favorite childhood meal. Then cook that meal. This will help start your collection of family tradition recipes.

84. VITAMIN K-2 - Kale, Collard Greens, Other Dark Leafy Greens

Vitamin K has three main components – K1, K2 and K3. Vitamin K1 has a big impact on proper blood clotting. Little is known about Vitamin K3. In this section I want to focus on Vitamin K2 which regulates when calcium ends up in the body. K2 plays a huge role in bone metabolism and there are a number of studies that suggest it helps prevent fractures and osteoporosis.

People that are deficient in Vitamin K have a much higher risk of bone fractures. This is especially true with senior citizens and is one of the contributing factors in their having higher rates of broken hips. Vitamin K regulates Osteoclasts which regulate bone demineralization. When the osteoclasts are allowed to run wild and unchecked, too much of the minerals are pulled from the bones and the bones become weak and brittle.

The K2 form of vitamin K is made within the body from K1 by your gut flora and other microorganisms. Because of this, you need to eat enough foods containing adequate amounts of Vitamin K1. The K1 form of Vitamin K is found in plant foods. This is required in order for green plants to conduct the photosynthesis process.

There is very little K2 that is found naturally in foods UNLESS they have been fermented or otherwise processed using bacteria or other microorganisms. So fermented foods, such as Tempeh and Miso contains substantial amounts of K2.

Where do you find large amounts of Vitamin K? Well you probably guessed it – Dark Leafy Greens, such as, Kale, Spinach, Watercress and Radicchio just to name a few. Kale has by far more vitamin K than any other food – giving you 6 times your daily requirement. So add Kale and Spinach to your daily diet to insure you have healthy bones.

ACTION ITEM: Here is another reason to add Kale and Spinach to your diet. This week try to have Kale in at least 4 meals. Add to salads, smoothies or mixed steamed vegetables.

85. BREAK-FAST! The Most Important Meal Of The Day

There is much debate about this important topic. There are plenty of research studies that support the long standing nutrition mantra 'breakfast is the most important meal of the day.' But at the same time there are new studies that tend to show that there really is not much difference between the two groups – the ones who eat breakfast and those who don't.

So here is my opinion –

If you are not eating breakfast and you feel great and your moods are stable then by all means continue skipping breakfast BUT if you are lacking in energy and you suffer from depression/anxiety or other mood disorders then start eating a 'healthy' breakfast.

If on the other hand you are eating a breakfast and feel crappy and your moods are in the dumps then try changing your breakfast to a healthier breakfast and see what happens. I suppose you can try skipping breakfast and see how you feel but I am willing to bet you that skipping breakfast will not help overcome your mood swings or depression.

Here are a few reasons why eating a healthy, well balanced breakfast will help improve your health and moods.

- It will provide you with plenty of energy for activities at work, school or play during the morning and helps prevent the mid-morning slump.
- You will have a jump start on getting enough vitamins, minerals and other important nutrients that your body needs every day.
- There is a tendency to eat more food than you usually do at the next meal, or you will munch on junk food to hold off hunger.
- Can cause or increase mid-morning cravings which can make losing weight more difficult.
- Eating one or two large meals can make you feel sluggish, tired and add to feelings of depression after the meal.

Tips on breakfast meals and preparation

- Smoothies are fairly quick and easy and very healthy. I make mine the night before for a quick 'grab and go' breakfast.
- Make an egg omelet with lots of your favorite veggies. To save time cut up the vegetables the night before.
- Try to include 2-3 different foods and include- A Protein, Vegetables, A Whole Grain and maybe you can add a little fruit.

You will be healthier, more efficient in most all you do and your moods will greatly improve by recharging your brain and body every morning. You recharge by eating a complete and healthy breakfast.

ACTION ITEM: Start eating a healthy breakfast every morning. Change from the junk cereal to Egg and Veggie Omelet and a slice of whole grain toast with real butter.

86. DETOX - Personal Care And Cleaners

Once you have detoxed your body it is very important that you keep new toxins from entering your body. One easy way is to detox your home of all the harmful chemicals that you may breath in or put on your body.

All the different toxins, if allowed in or on your body, can create chaos and disorder within your body, your biochemistry and even your cellular health. Don't forget about some of the negative effects they can have on the environment.

These harmful chemicals are called endocrine disruptors, and they can 'disrupt' the hormones and especially those that keep your metabolism running right. You might be able to cut down on chemical overloaded process foods but this may not be enough. You need to remove the harmful toxins from your HOME also.

Harmful toxins can be found in your household cleaning products, personal care products and make-up products. By swapping out these products with more natural based products will go a long ways towards improving your over-all health. Your metabolism, moods and wellness will get a well-deserved boost.

Here are the first three areas in your home to start with:

- Make-Up, Personal Care and Beauty Supplies such as shampoo, deodorant, toothpaste, mouthwash, etc. These are a major source of 'chemicals' that can be toxic to your body. You can find such toxins as lead, mercury, toluene, parabens, formaldehyde, and phthalates, just to name a few. There are more and more 'all natural' brands of make-up and personal care lines on the market.

- Household Cleaners – These chemical-based cleaners are exposing you to many harsh and poisonous substances. Some of the worst ones are the drain cleaners, oven cleaners and toilet bowl cleaners. You can easily change to all Natural Cleaners such as white vinegar, castile soap, lemon juice, baking soda, etc. Sometimes just plain water will clean something good enough. There are also a lot of companies that are starting to market 'environmentally' friendly cleaners and soaps.

- Another common source of toxins in the home is artificial room deodorizers! These spray product contain VOC's (volatile organic compounds) that are sprayed into the air you breathe. These VOCs can cause drowsiness, headaches, nausea, and dizziness and can impair memory and moods. Use natural products like essential oils to freshen up your rooms.

These are just a few of the places you can start to detox your home. Your body, brain will feel great and your moods will soar once you detox your home and your body. Make it a priority to detox your home first and then detox your body. Your overall health will improve.

ACTION ITEM: This week find two toxic products in your home and replace them with a non-toxic version. Then the following week replace another and then another.

87. SLEEP - 7 to 8 Continuous Hours

If you want to reach your goal of having a healthy, energetic, and happy life you must get enough sleep. Enough sleep is 7 to 8 hours every night. These must be continuous hours as much as possible.

During sleep your body and especially your brain works hard to detox. This is a time when the body rests and during this resting period your brain has a chance to unwind and go through a detox period and filing memories into the long term files. Studies have shown that when you are deficient in Vitamin S (Sleep) you will have problems making good decisions, coping with change and controlling emotions. The lack of sleep has been linked to depression and suicide.

Here are a few quick tips on getting a better night sleep. All are simple and easy BUT they all might entail some lifestyle changes. So try some of these tips:

- o   Try to maintain a night time schedule, go to bed and get up about the same time, even on the weekends. This will help keep the body clock in rhythm. Sleeping in on the weekends is like going on and off 'Daylight Savings Time' once a week!
- o   Make the hour before bed a time to unwind and make it your quiet time. Do not do strenuous exercise, watch

t.v. or use other electronics as the artificial light is known to affect the brain and makes falling asleep harder.

- o Avoid alcohol and large meals within a couple of hours of going to bed.
- o Avoid caffeine drinks and cigarettes at night. Caffeine can stay in your system for 8 hours.
- o Do some sort of relaxation technique before bed, such as meditation or listen to a guided meditation CD. This is my technique of choice. You can try a hot bath also.

You need to find what works for you. You MUST find ways to get 8 hours of sleep every night for a healthy, happy and prosperous life. Your moods will greatly improve also.

ACTION ITEM: This week try one of the above suggestions and see if you don't sleep better and longer. Settle for nothing less than 7 hours and preferably 8 hours of sleep a night.

88.   CANDY: Buy 1 Piece At A Time - Never Buy A Box Or Bag

This is a sweet and short little secret. On occasion, when you want to have a sweet little treat just buy 1 piece at a time. Do not buy a whole bag or box and take them home! Repeat – only buy 1 peace at a time. You know if you buy a whole bag or box of candy and take it home you will eat all of them. This also holds true with cookies, donuts etc.

89. CHIPS: Only On National Holidays Or When Scooping Up Healthy Salsa or Dip

Chips and Dips have gone together for 50 years. They are part of the foundation of the Standard American Diet (SAD) along with Hamburger, Hotdogs and French Fries. Chips and all variations are a highly processed factory food.

All the different variation of chips is nothing more that the starchy portion of a vegetable or grain, fried in refined oils with added salt and flavoring. Some may be baked or popped and have sea salt sprinkled on them but they are all highly processed and do not contain much real nutrition.

Here is a list of the nutritional value from a handful (28 grams) of chips. The different types of chips vary but they are generally about the same – Calories: 140, Oxidized Seed Oil: 6-10 grams, Refined Carbohydrates: 16-20 grams and a dose of salt, no vitamins or minerals.

These foods seem to be fairly inexpensive but in reality they are not. These different chips range from about $3 a pound to $6 a pound. The best buy is home cooked popcorn.

So here is the real tip. Make eating chips a national holiday treat and only eat them with a healthy, homemade salsa or dip.

ACTION ITEM: Cut out all the different type of chips from your daily diet and only eat them on National Holidays and only with a healthy dip or salsa.

90.   LEGUMES: 5-6 Days A Week

Legumes are seeds that split in half. Some of the more common edible legumes are beans, peas, lentils, peanuts and soybeans. These seeds are a great source of fiber and protein plus a wealth of other beneficial nutrients. Because legumes have the ability to pull nitrogen from the atmosphere, which is important part of the different amino acids, they are among the best plant based protein sources.

Legumes are a great source of healthy fibers. These healthy fibers consist of soluble fibers and resistant starch. These fibers pass through the stomach and small intestines undigested until they get to the colon or large intestines. Here they become food for the friendly bacteria and microbiome that live there. You need a healthy gut and in order to have a healthy gut you must keep the friendly bacteria well fed and happy.

These soluble fibers and resistant starches will help keep you feeling full, which will reduce the amount of food you eat and can help you lose weight in the long run.

Another great reason to consume legumes is because they are very cheap. They are one of the best foods where you get the most nutritional value for your money.

There is a down side to these foods – they also contain some negative or anti – nutrients, which if eaten in large quantities can impair your health in certain cases. The good news is that there are ways to help neutralize these anti-nutrients by using traditional methods of preparing these legumes such as – soaking, boiling, sprouting or fermenting.

Worth noting – If you currently have depression / anxiety AND you normally DO NOT eat legumes then try adding them into your diet and see if the depression improves. But if you currently are suffering from depression and you have a fair amount of Legumes in your daily diet, try removing Legumes from your diet and see if your depression symptoms lessen. Some research suggests people who have intolerance to beans and legumes also have depression. Experiment with Legumes.

Bottom line – most people need to include properly prepared, legumes 5-6 times a week as part of a well-balanced, real food diet. You will start to feel healthier and happier in no time.

ACTION ITEM: This week add legumes into 3 meals. Try several different varieties and start off with smaller portions and then gradually increase frequency.

91. FRUIT: In Season And As Fresh As Possible. Frozen Work!

When it comes to eating fruit, keep these two things in mind – Eat the fruit as fresh as possible and when they are in season. The next best thing is frozen fruit. Frozen fruit may be more preferable in some cases. Frozen fruit is ripe when picked and then quickly frozen. Most nutrients are still there in large quantities.

Fruit you purchase in the stores, if not in season, have been picked earlier and put in storage to be sold in stores later. These do not have near the amount of nutrients as those picked and eaten fresh. So eat fruit in season, fresh or frozen.

Since fruit come from plants, they are REAL, WHOLE foods. They are not highly processed junk foods. We have been eating fruit for thousands of years. Some people consider fruits as 'nature's fast food' because you can just grab and go. There is very little preparation time and some come in their own package.

Here is a short list of reason you want to eat 2-3 servings of fruit each day:

- Very Filling or Satiating – Because of all the fiber, water content and all the chewing you feel full and actually will eat less of the other foods. Look for fruit with the highest fiber, vitamins and minerals and with less sugar and calories.
- High in Vitamins and Minerals - such as Vitamin C, Potassium and Folate. Many people are deficient in Folate and Potassium. Let's not forget all the other various antioxidants and phytonutrients found in fruits.
- Natural Fructose – Yes fruit has fructose but it is found in small quantities and it is easily tolerated because it takes more chewing to eat the fruit and is slower to digest.

Because different fruits contain different nutrients and amounts make sure you eat a variety of fruits. Try a different fruit each week. Don't be afraid of some of the more exotic ones. Here is a list of a few of the top fruits based on nutritional content:

Berries – Blueberries, Raspberries, Strawberries, Blackberries, Gooseberries (Goji), Cranberries

Watermelon, Lemons, Grapefruit, Guavas

Higher in sugar – Apples, Banana's, Pineapples, Cherries, Mango and Oranges

Remember to eat 2-3 servings of fruit every day. Get them as fresh as possible and remember frozen fruit is good, especially in smoothies.

ACTION ITEM: This week try several different fruits, especially berries. Berries top the list of some of the most nutritious fruits.

92.   SEEDS And NUTS - Variety: Eat A Handful Every Day

Nuts and seeds are very nutritious and tasty. More and more research shows that seeds and nuts help balance your moods and give your brain a powerful boost. So if you want to think clearer and/or give your moods a boost then munch on nuts and seeds. Eat a variety and just a handful or so is all you need.

They all seem to help your nervous system to become healthier, which means you feel happier and your thinking is clearer. According to a Reader's Digest article "Fight Back With Foods" the under-consumption or deficiency in Omega-3 fatty acids can lead some people into depression. Your brain and central nervous system needs the following nutrients to function properly – Omega-3's, Vitamin E, Vitamin B6, Magnesium, Tryptophan, Phosphatidyl-choline and Choline.

We are talking about common nuts and seeds and some of the more exotic seeds and nuts. They all seem to work well in clearing up 'brain fog' and feeling happier and healthier. Let's take a quick look at some of the seeds and nuts and find out why they help your brain and moods.

Walnuts: They are an excellent source of nutrients for your brain. They contain a good amount of the Vitamins E and B6. Their contents are 15 to 20 percent Protein. They contain Linoleic Acid (Omega-6 fatty acids) and Alpha-linoleic acids (Omega-3 fatty acids).

Cashew Nuts: These nuts are high in magnesium which helps to open up blood vessels in the brain which allows more oxygen-rich blood to flow to and through the brain.

Almonds: They are an excellent source of Phenylalanine which is vital for proper brain function and neurological health.

Pecans and Peanuts: Both of these nuts provide the brain with Choline, another vital nutrient for the brain. It is needed in ample amounts for healthy brain development and proper memory functions.

Flax Seeds: These little seeds are a great source of the mood-boosting Omega-3 fatty acids. These are a great replacement for those who do not like eating fish.

Pumpkin Seeds: High in Tryptophan. Eating a handful a day is a safe and natural way to reduce mild insomnia and depression.

Sunflower Seeds: Also high in tryptophan along with thiamine (a vitamin b) both are great for cognitive function and improved memory.

One of the most important nutrients for the brain, a major structural and functional component of the brain-cell membrane is Phosphatidyl-choline. If you are depleted in this, your brain cells will start to degenerate and die. Your body needs choline and lecithin to produce Phosphatidyl-choline. You need choline to produce acetylcholine which is a major player in maintaining good memory.

The good news is that nuts contain a good supply of choline and lecithin so your body can produce Phosphatidyl-choline and Acetylcholine for a healthy brain and good memory. Eat a handful of nuts daily and also eat a variety of nuts. Hundreds of studies have been done to support this secret.

Note: Tree nuts are on the Food Intolerance List because some people have intolerance to tree nuts or peanuts. If you suffer from a mood disorder and have no clear reason and you eat nuts on a regular basis, try to remove them from your diet and see if the depression symptoms clear up.

ACTION ITEMS: Include a handful of nuts in your daily diet and also include a variety, unless of course you have a known allergy or intolerance for peanuts and tree nuts.

93. HEALTHY DESSERTS: Minimize Sugar - Use Winter Fruits

Everyone loves a nice dessert after dinner. The problem is most desserts contain tons of added sugar. So here is a great tip – trade those highly processed, sugar laden desserts in for those with less sugar and use more Winter Fruits.

Fruit is considered nature's candy. Most are sweet and great tasting. Leave a bowl of fresh fruit and a bowl of fresh vegetables on a table and see which bowl is taken from the most. It will always be the fruit.

According to most lists out there the following fruits will be listed as winter fruits –

Apples – most varieties
Bananas
Citrus Fruit – grapefruit, tangelos, clementine and all varieties of oranges
Grapes
Kiwi
Pears
Lemons

Here are a few dessert ideas using winter fruits, keep the added sugars to a minimum –

Apple Crisp topped with homemade Granola – there are a lot of recipes available for both the apple crisp and the granola.

Fruit dipped in Dark Chocolate or melted Cacao – Winter Strawberries need to be dressed up a little and chocolate works great for that. Here is a great little video on how to dress strawberries in chocolate.
http://www.marthastewart.com/313844/chocolate-covered-strawberries

Baked Apple – Apples are plentiful and delicious. Baking an apple is simple, easy and tasty. Here is a popular recipe -
http://simplyrecipes.com/recipes/baked_apples/

Tropical Fruit Delight – Mix chunks of ripe pineapple with slices of banana with grated coconut. Feel free to add in other tropical fruit like sliced kiwi.

Banana Nut Bread – There are tons of recipes available. Here are a couple of tips to make a healthier version of the bread. Replace ½ of the white flour with whole wheat flour or other whole grain flour. Cut the sugar by 1/3 and use brown sugar instead of the white sugar and use real butter instead of the less healthy oils normally called out in recipes. Don't forget to double the amount of walnuts.

Bottom line: In the winter, when you have that strong craving for a dessert after dinner, please think fruit and make it the main ingredient. When you make healthier choices your body, mind and moods will feel healthier and more alive.

ACTION ITEM: This week, reach for a piece of fruit or fruit filled dish when you want to help satisfy the 'after dinner dessert' craving.

94. SUPPLEMENTS - Amino Acids - Food For Moods

When it comes to brain health and happiness Amino Acids are one of the key nutrients. There are other important nutrients but Amino acids are a major key in regulating moods. If you are suffering from symptoms of depression or anxiety, chances are really high that you are deficient in one or more amino acids. Let's take a quick peak at why this is the case.

Neurotransmitter molecules carry neural impulses around inside each of your brain's nerve cells. There are dozens of different kinds of neurotransmitters, each with their own important function. Out of these dozens, I just want to touch on 3 of these neurotransmitters:

Dopamine
Norepinephrine
Serotonin

These three are part of a class of chemicals called monoamines. These monoamines are critical in maintaining normal moods. They come into play in our experiences regarding fear and pleasure. Researchers also believe that many of your cognitive functions, like learning, memory and attention (concentration) are influenced by these monoamines.

Depression, ADHD, and Anxiety can be caused by the imbalance or disruption of these neurotransmitters. It is vitally important that you minimize these disruptions or deficiencies of these neurotransmitters by providing your body the needed associated Amino Acids. Let's take a quick look at which amino acids affect these neurotransmitters.

The body takes the amino acids that are found in your protein foods and converts them into the monoamine neurotransmitters. For example:

Phenylalanine is the amino acid that is converted into **Dopamine**

Tyrosine is needed to make **Noreprinephrine** (Noradrenaline)

Tryptophan is the amino acid that is needed to be converted into **5-HTP** which is converted into **Serotonin**. Tryptophan (found in food – not available as a supplement) is converted into 5-HTP (not found in food – is available as a supplement) is converted into Serotonin.

As you can see it is very important to get enough of all the different amino acids for a healthy brain and to overcome depression, anxiety and other mood disorders. Normally you can get enough of all the different amino-acids **IF** you are eating a healthy, well-balanced diet.

According to researchers, nutrition is one of the major contributors to your health and well-being including proper brain functions and moods. Many of the food patterns you experience during depression are the same ones that precede depression and other mood disorders. These include skipping meals, craving and eating sweet sugary foods, poor appetite and poor food choices.

Just like other important nutrients such as minerals, vitamins, and omega-3 it is a good idea to supplement your diet with Amino Acids. Researchers and Clinicians have found that taking an Amino Acid supplement have reduced symptoms of depression and help elevate moods. Researchers are doing more and more studies in the area of epigenetics (DNA-Gene expression) using amino acid supplement to help control different mood and brain disorders. The findings are very promising.

If you want a healthy brain and a happier disposition try taking an Amino Acid supplement. In the meantime try up grading your diet also. You will be glad you did.

ACTION ITEM: This week try taking an Amino Acid supplement and see if you can feel a little less stressed, calmer and happier.

95. JOIN OR FORM A NUTRITION AND COOKING CLUB - ON OR OFFLINE

Why would this be listed as one of the top 101 Secrets to Health and Happiness? Well it's very simple. In order to eat healthy you have to know how to cook healthy foods. You need great recipes, experience working with different kitchen appliances, etc.

A cooking or nutrition club is a group of people, friends or neighbors who get together on a semi-regular or regular time frame to cook together. Sometimes you want to cook a large batch of food for freezing or storage but you don't want to do all the work yourself. This is a great way to learn how to cook foods that you are not familiar with. It is a time to have fun together.

Maybe someone in your group is an expert at making bread and you want to learn how to bake bread. The bread making expert can teach the group how to make bread and you all share in bringing the ingredients.

Maybe a member is an expert at using a specific piece of equipment so you all gather to learn how to use that equipment. Or what if a member owns an expensive or unusual piece of cooking equipment, such as a sausage maker and you all get together and makes sausage.

Maybe the best reason is just get together and have fun while learning or improving your cooking skills, sharing recipes and enjoying the finished product together. You can even explore different healthy ethnic foods that you have never tried before. It is always fun and more enjoyable to learn as a group and from each other.

ACTION ITEM: ***Find a cooking club either in your area or one online and join it. IF you can't find one in your area, start one. There are a number of great websites that can give you tips on how to start and run a cooking club in your neighborhood.***

96. NIGHTSHADE VEGETABLES - Healthy For You, Maybe

Nightshade fruits and vegetables are nutritious and beneficial for most people. However, there are some people who have a sensitivity or intolerance with this group of foods, and are unable to fully digest them. Sensitivity may cause you to have symptoms of bloating, gas, nausea, and diarrhea. They can cause pain in the joints, headaches and symptoms of depression.

If you are suffering from any of the symptoms listed above you might try removing all nightshade foods from your diet for 30 days to see how you feel. If these symptoms clear-up then you know you have to avoid all nightshade foods.

Which foods fall into the nightshade category?

Potatoes – We are talking about white, red, blue-skinned and yellow varieties. Know that Sweet potatoes and Yams are NOT nightshade foods.

Tomatoes – This includes all tomatoes varieties, raw and cooked and this includes foods made from tomatoes, like ketchup, sauces and pastes.

Peppers – Bell Peppers, Cayenne Peppers, Jalapenos and Paprika to name a few. This would include any spice made from peppers such as Paprika and dried peppers.

Eggplants – These are fairly easy to avoid. Eggplants are used in various ethnic dishes such as Thai, Indian, and Italian. Eggplant Parmesan is one of the more well-known dishes.

Goji Berries – Since these are not all that common in our western diet, they are fairly easy to avoid. But these nutritious little berries are becoming more common in juices, smoothies and different nutritional supplements, so read the labels carefully.

Again, these foods are delicious and very nutritious for most people. Just be aware that if you suffer from depression, joint pains, or from digestive issues nightshade foods might be the cause and it is worth eliminating them from diet and then seeing how you feel.

If you find that you are NOT sensitive to nightshade foods make sure you try to incorporate them into your daily or weekly diet as they do contain a great amount of healthy vitamins, minerals and other nutrients.

ACTION ITEM: Experiment with nightshade fruits and vegetables. If you are eating them and your health is not where you want it to be try removing them from your diet and see if you look and feel better.

If you are not eating nightshade foods and feel like you need a boost, add them to your diet and see if you feel better.

97. STOCK-BASED VEGETABLE SOUPS
- Homemade - Once A Week

Vegetable broths are a very healthy and versatile part of any diet. These broths are delicious, contain tons of minerals and will help alkalize your body and keep it from getting too acidic. Both vegetable and bone broths have been part of the human diet for thousands of years.

Broths and soups have been used almost as a medicine. Remember when you were a child and got a cold. I will bet your mom gave you chicken noodle soup or a vegetable broth. Vegetable broths are commonly incorporated into different cleanses or detoxes. Broths are used to heal the gut.

The tasty vegetable broths warms, soothes and nourishes the body. It has healing properties and help with;

- Boosting the immune system
- Brain health
- Joint pain and overall joint health
- Digestion issues
- Over all skin and body health

Vegetable broth can be used straight and sipped like a tea, as base for soups or sauces. It is great to use in place of water when cooking quinoa, rice and kasha (buckwheat). It adds more flavor as well as additional nutrition.

You can make vegetable broth from most any vegetables, but if you want to make a broth that has a deep flavor and immune boosting properties use the following vegetables:

- Shitake mushrooms or any other mushrooms

- Garlic
- Ginger
- Turmeric and
- Kombu or any other seaweed

For a wonderful and nutritious vegetable soup stock recipe check out this one:

http://gourmandeinthekitchen.com/2014/detox-vegetable-broth-recipe/

Now that you have made the vegetable stock you can use it to make any dish that calls for soup stock. You can also make great vegetable soups using this vegetable stock as the base. Vegetable soups are really healthy and nutritious. Soups help soothe the body, mind and spirit. Try having a bowl full of vegetable soup or broth on a weekly basis and your body and mind will feel wonderful. It will also help keep the common cold away.

ACTION ITEM: This week try making a simple vegetable soup stock. Then drink it like a tea and use it to cook with to add additional flavor to your dishes.

98. HERBS AND SPICES: Use For Flavoring And Healing

"Studies show that many different herbs and spices offer health benefits," so says David Heber, Director of the UCLA Center for Human Nutrition.

"We're now starting to see a scientific basis for why people have been using spices medicinally for thousands of years," says

Bharat Aggarwal, Ph.D., professor at the University Of Texas M.D. Anderson Cancer Center in Houston.

Not only do herbs and spices add flavor to your food dishes but they also have many health and healing properties. Because of this it is important to your overall health to include many different herbs and spices in your food preparations. Let's take a look of at a few herbs and spices and their health benefits.

Sage: Sipping on sage tea is great for upset stomachs and sore throats. Studies have shown that spraying sore throats with a sage solution (sage tea) gives effective pain relief.

Chili Peppers: According to studies, the pungent compound in hot chilies – Capsaicin, helps to increase the body's metabolism and helps boost fat burning.

Ginger: Helps soothe an upset stomach, nausea, fights common colds and reduces arthritis pain. Throughout history ginger has been used in treating stomach troubles.

Rosemary: In a recent study individuals achieved higher scores on memory and alertness tests after piping in a mist of aromatic rosemary oil into their study rooms. Rosemary garlands were used by the ancient Greek scholars when they studied to help them remember.

Cinnamon: The ancient Romans, Greeks and King Solomon highly prized cinnamon and used it to relieve stomach problems and to boost appetite. Today it is used to stabilize blood sugar levels of Type 2 diabetics.

Parsley: This herb contains anti-cancer properties. Researchers at the University of Missouri have shown that parsley can actually prevent breast cancer-cell growth.

Turmeric: Turmeric is made into a paste and then it is applied to wounds to speed up healing, in India. They also treat the common cold and other respiratory problems with a turmeric tea.

Saffron: In Persian traditional medicine, saffron is used to uplift moods, and is made into a medicinal tea. They also use saffron in the preparation of rice dishes. Saffron has been used to relieve symptoms of PMS.

These are just a few of the very healthy and tasty herbs and spices. As spices, they all can help transform a dull and tasteless food into a very delicious dish. The great side effect of cooking with spices is it just may improve your health, mood and memory. Start adding spices into your daily food dishes. Don't forget to make and drink herbal teas when you are not feeling well.

ACTION ITEM: This week experiment different herbs and spices when cooking. Try making and drinking an herbal tea and see if you don't feel better.

99. SUPER FOODS FROM AROUND THE WORLD

There are many different foods that have been used not only by ancient civilizations but also in modern times that are extremely healthy and beneficial but are still under-utilized here in the United States.

If you add some of these foods into your daily and weekly diet you will notice a profound difference. Since it is very difficult to get these foods fresh here in the United States they are usually consumed as a powder or dried. Let's take a quick look at several of these healthy superfoods from around the world.

Acai Berry - This can be easily found as a juice. Acai juice is super high in Anthocyanin, which researchers at Texas A&M, say will greatly increase the blood antioxidant levels because it is a potent antioxidant.

Goji Berries – For hundreds and even thousands of years Goji Berries have been used in Chinese herbal medicine and is commonly used in herbal tea and tonic drinks. These tasty berries are a potent source of Vitamin C and especially beta-carotene. They also contain 13% protein and are high in iron which helps to build up the blood. Goji berries also help to keep the liver and kidneys healthy and in shape and great for those who are anemic and need extra iron.

I just love adding a few of these healthy dried berries into my homemade trail mix, and refrigerator oatmeal. I even have a few plants in my garden.

Cacao or Dark Chocolate - In the ancient America's, the Incas considered a drink made from cacao as 'the drink of the gods'. Cacao is available as a powder for making drinks and smoothies or as 'nibs' (chunks of roasted cacao) which are a crunchy treat.

Cacao contains Anandamide which is a mood improver and is known as the 'bliss' molecule. It helps create a feeling of euphoria. In other words it helps balance mood swings. It does this by helping to boost brain levels of the neurotransmitter – Serotonin, the feel good brain hormone. Studies have shown that cacao boosts the brain levels of calming hormones and helps restore a sense of well-being and happiness.

Maca – is a tuber (large radish like) that is grown at the higher elevation of the South American Andes Mountains. This plant has been used for centuries as an adaptogen (it helps anywhere within the body where it is needed).

It is critically important in this stress filled world that we all live in, that you include a food like Maca into your diet as it is known to increase the body's resistance to fatigue, stress factors, anxiety and trauma.

Camu Camu – this Amazon fruit is known for its extremely high Vitamin C and antioxidant that is responsible for boosting immune system, neutralizing the damaging effects of those pesky free radicals and preventing oxidative stress in the body.

The Vitamin C in Camu Camu is powerful, natural and better utilized by the body than the Ascorbic Acid used in many vitamin supplements. Because of this, the Camu Camu Vitamin C, according to researchers, is one of the best nutrients for the brain, the central nervous system, skin and eyes and very useful in making certain neurotransmitters needed for ideal brain function. A healthy brain = healthy moods.

As you can see, there are some foods from other areas of the world that have some tremendous health benefits that you can try. These are found at most health food stores and online. Experiment with some of these tasty super foods from around the world and see for yourself why they have been used for hundreds and even thousands of years by the Chinese and the ancient people of South America.

ACTION ITEM: This week go to your local health food store and buy some Maca, Cacao or dried Goji berries. Add to smoothies or trail mix. Research and experiment with these amazing foods.

100. BONE BROTH - The Other Elixir Of Life

There are many people who consider bone broth as –"The Other or Second Elixir of Life" behind water. Bone Broth can be used in place of water when cooking or just sipped as a tea. Either way, bone broth is very nutritious, healthy and delicious.

Bone broths have the following health benefits;

- High in Calcium, Magnesium and Phosphorus – great for building healthy and strong bones and teeth
    - Women who drink bone broth have babies with stronger and healthier bones
- High in Collagen
    - Helps remove wrinkles and cellulite
    - Lubricates the joints and helps with joint pain
    - Heals leaky gut problems and aids in digestion
- High In Amino Acid Glycerin
    - Supports better sleep
    - Aids the liver in detoxifying your body

How to make bone broth

Bone broth is made by boiling bones from healthy animals. This process pulls out the minerals, collagen and glycerin from the bones. Bones can be from beef, bison, fish, lamb and poultry, which ever ones you like to eat.

Steps to make bone broth
1. Blanch Bones – Boil bones for 20 minutes
2. Roach Bones – Roast at 450 degrees. Roast until the point of being 'too done'
3. Using a larger pot than you think you will need, add bones, little garlic, onion and black pepper and cover with lots of water
4. Simmer – Up to 24 hours for best flavor (unless using poultry then a few hours will due)
5. Strain out solids and Cool Quickly – add Ice and put in fridge.

There are a lot of recipes on the internet but for the best results keep ingredients to a minimum. Try bone broth and enjoy the health benefits that it can provide.

ACTION ITEM: This week either make your own homemade bone broth or pick some up at your local health food store. Homemade always tastes better and you know what you are getting.

101. SULFUR - The Forgotten Mineral

Before you go wrinkling up or pinching your nose, I am not talking about the yellow stinky mineral that is mined or found in smelly sulfur springs. I am talking about the other Sulfur – the organic version that humans are absolutely dependent on for a healthy body and mind.

This sulfur is formally called MethylSulfonyMethane or more commonly called MSM. The term Organic Sulfur and MSM is the same thing and are commonly used interchangeably. Organic Sulfur is known for some pretty amazing health benefits. MSM is a critical mineral that is needed by every cell in your body. Organic Sulfur is needed for over 140 functions or to make compounds needed in your body. It is the 3rd most plentiful mineral in your body.

When was the last time you heard any doctor talk about Sulfur and the need to get enough of this mineral into your body? Very few people are talking about sulfur but they should be!

There are only 2 ways to get sulfur – Supplements and Foods. The problem is - in today's food there is very little sulfur, even in the sulfur rich foods. So the best way to get the sulfur you need is through supplementation.

Reasons why you should be taking organic sulfur –

- sulfur enables the transport of oxygen across cell membranes so the cells can regenerate efficiently
- Reduces joint inflammation and pain
- Supports the creation of insulin – reduces the need for insulin for diabetics

- Heals skin issues and promotes healthy and young looking skin
- Transports nutrients into the cells
- Needed in liver and cell regeneration
- The list goes on and on.................

Because most of us have an organic sulfur deficiency, we all have health issues. People who take the organic sulfur report improvements in nearly every area of the body. Allergies go away, cataracts disappear, skin issues clear up, muscle and joint pains are gone, and on and on. It almost looks like a miracle supplement. My wife's coworkers comment on how good her face looks and how much younger see looks. They want to know her secret.

Organic Sulfur is the forgotten mineral but I strongly suggest that if you have some health issues you might just want to try taking MSM supplementation for 90 days and see if you don't feel better. It has no side effects and it is difficult to take too much. Try it and see what happens. It just might make you look and feel like a totally new and younger person.

ACTION ITEM: This week try taking Organic Sulfur (MSM) supplement. For the best results take it in either Crystal or powdered form, mixed in warm, filtered water. Remember – it may not taste great but it is great for the body.

THE SUMMARY

As you finish reading this book I sincerely hope that you have found these tips helpful and enlightening. None of these tips were deep secrets from some far away Tibetan Monk or a book from some recently discovered civilization. They are simple everyday things you can do in your daily life.

Many of these 'secrets' were things you probably did as a child growing up. I can promise you that if you will take these tips serious **_and implement them into your life_**, by doing the action items; your life will become healthier, happier and more peaceful.

You have learned that there are Primary Foods and Secondary Foods and that each of them play an important role in your health and happiness. You have learned that you cannot neglect either.

Neglect the Primary Foods and your stress level will go off the charts. Having great relationships with your spouse, children, parents, friends and co-workers is a must if you are to overcome symptoms of depression and anxiety. Having great relationships will come in handy when you do have some of those re-occurring down days.

Exercising and being active can, for some people, be the main thing that eliminates depression. Being active and exercising can be just as effective as medications. So get up and get moving!

The ideal situation is to be in a career or job that you love. This may not be that realistic for most people but it is possible. But what you can do is change a few things at your current job so that you can enjoy it more. Stress at work must be minimized if you are to ever defeat depression.

Let's not forget Spirituality. Hopefully you will take time to think about your spirituality and what spirituality means to you. Once you know, do something every day to feed that spirituality. Having this in your life will help you overcome and deal with trials that may come up in your life.

As you may well know, STRESS KILLS! There are some great tips here on how to manage and deal with stress. Try some of the deep breathing exercises, learn some Qi Gong movements or implement guided visualization into your daily or weekly routine. Try to eliminate some of the sources of stress. Regardless of how successful you are at removing stress from your life, you must learn how to manage and deal with your stress.

Now let's review some of the tips concerning the Secondary Foods. For many people, including you, the sources of their depression or anxiety symptoms may be from food intolerance or sensitivity. For this group of individuals finding out which foods, such as dairy or gluten, that they are intolerant of and removing them from their diet is all they have to do and the symptoms disappear.

Your brain needs all the nutrients it can get so chew your food well. Digestion starts in the mouth and the more you chew your food the easier and more complete the digestion is when it hits the stomach. Eating home cooked meals with your family is something that is becoming lost in our society. Use healthy foods to get the family together to help strengthen family relationships.

You now have 101 great ideas on being a healthier and happier person but you have to take the first step and keep taking steps thereafter. These are easy, little steps, not giant leaps out of your comfort zone. It all begins with the first step and taking the next step – no matter what! You can do it - because I believe in YOU!

RESOURCES:

Here is couple of resources that are available to you. Feel free to check them out and use them as you see fit.

DEPRESSION TO HAPPINESS – The 100 Day Challenge
Creator – Timothy Baumann, CHC

This is a 100 day challenge that will change your entire life IF you are ready and willing to put forth the needed effort. In the book and challenge we go into more details on many of the tips contained within this book. It includes 14 weekly emails with action items – similar to the ones in this book. The Challenge contains a complete 14 day detox, an elimination diet (to look for and find food intolerances) and a complete 28 day clean eating plan plus much more.

This is for those who are serious about regaining their health and/or overcoming depression, anxiety or other mood disorders.

There are two options within this 100 day challenge. You can choose between The DIY (Do It Yourself) version and the Group Coaching version. The Group Coaching is for those who want and need more support and encouragement.

For more information –
www.depressiontohappiness.com/the100daychallenge

Qsciences - EMPowerplus Q96 and other supplements

These are the supplements that my wife and I take. They have 20 years of history and over 26 independent studies done by top universities and researchers. Specifically formulated and designed for the brain. The company also has all the great supplements discussed earlier.

Information: www.brainsupplementsite.com Or www.14166.myqsciences.com/products.aspx

BOOK

NUTRIENT POWER – Heal Your Biochemistry and Heal Your Brain by William J Walsh, PhD

SUPPORT

This is a closed group that is open for those who have purchased this book and for those who participate in the 100 Day Challenge listed above.

https://www.facebook.com/groups/depressiontohappiness/

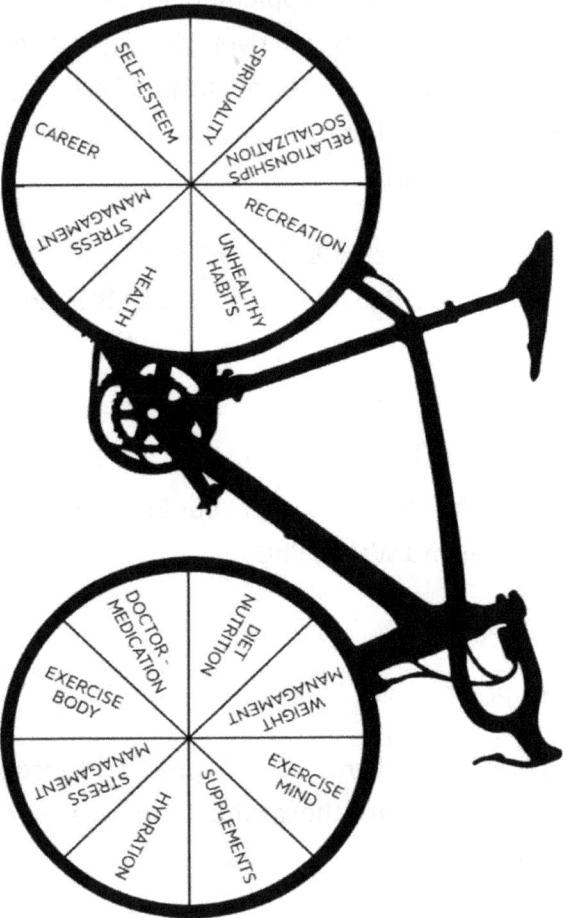

LIFE: PRIMARY WHEEL

- SELF-ESTEEM
- SPIRITUALITY
- CAREER
- RELATIONSHIPS SOCIALIZATION
- STRESS MANAGAMENT
- RECREATION
- HEALTH
- UNHEALTHY HABITS

HEALTH: SECONDARY WHEEL

- DOCTOR- MEDICATION
- NUTRITION
- DIET
- EXERCISE BODY
- WEIGHT MANAGAMENT
- STRESS MANAGAMENT
- EXERCISE MIND
- HYDRATION
- SUPPLEMENTS

www.ingramcontent.com/pod-product-compliance
Lightning Source LLC
Chambersburg PA
CBHW060924040426
42445CB00011B/772